Recent Results in Cancer Research

Fortschritte der Krebsforschung

Progrès dans les recherches sur le cancer

43

Nomenclature, Methodology and Results of Clinical Trials in Acute Leukemias

Edited by

G. Mathé · P. Pouillart · L. Schwarzenberg

With 79 Figures

Springer-Verlag Berlin Heidelberg New York 1973

Workshop held June 19 and 20, 1972 at the Centre National de la Recherche Scientifique (C.N.R.S.), 15, quai Anatole France, 75007 Paris, France

co-sponsored by

Institut de Cancérologie et d'Immunogénétique (I.C.I.G.)
Institut National de la Santé et de la Recherche Médicale (I.N.S.E.R.M.)
European Organization for Research on Treatment of Cancer (E.O.R.T.C.)
National Cancer Institute (N.C.I.)

Sponsored by the Swiss League against Cancer

ISBN-13:978-3-642-80778-7 e-ISBN-13:978-3-642-80776-3
DOI: 10.1007/978-3-642-80776-3

Nomenclature, Methodology and Results of Clinical Trials in Acute Leukemias

Edited by

G. Mathé · P. Pouillart · L. Schwarzenberg

With 79 Figures

Springer-Verlag New York Heidelberg Berlin 1973

Workshop held June 19 and 20, 1972 at the Centre National de la Recherche Scientifique (C.N.R.S.), 15, quai Anatole France, 75007 Paris, France

co-sponsored by

Institut de Cancérologie et d'Immunogénétique (I.C.I.G.)
Institut National de la Santé et de la Recherche Médicale (I.N.S.E.R.M.)
European Organization for Research on Treatment of Cancer (E.O.R.T.C.)
National Cancer Institute (N.C.I.)

Sponsored by the Swiss League against Cancer

ISBN-13:978-3-642-80778-7 e-ISBN-13:978-3-642-80776-3
DOI: 10.1007/978-3-642-80776-3

Nomenclature, Methodology and Results of Clinical Trials in Acute Leukemias

Edited by

G. Mathé · P. Pouillart · L. Schwarzenberg

With 79 Figures

1973
William Heinemann Medical Books Ltd., London
Springer-Verlag Berlin · Heidelberg · New York

Workshop held June 19 and 20, 1972 at the Centre National de la Recherche Scientifique (C.N.R.S.), 15, quai Anatole France, 75007 Paris, France

co-sponsored by

Institut de Cancérologie et d'Immunogénétique (I.C.I.G.)
Institut National de la Santé et de la Recherche Médicale (I.N.S.E.R.M.)
European Organization for Research on Treatment of Cancer (E.O.R.T.C.)
National Cancer Institute (N.C.I.)

Sponsored by the Swiss League against Cancer

ISBN-13:978-3-642-80778-7 e-ISBN-13:978-3-642-80776-3
DOI: 10.1007/978-3-642-80776-3

Contents

Third Session — Actuarial Results

List of Participants

AMIEL, J. L., Unité Fred-Siguier de Dévelopment Therapeutique, Institut de Cancérologie et d'Immunogénétique, Hôpital Paul-Brousse, 14—16, Avenue Paul-Vaillant-Couturier, 94800 Villejuif, France

AUR, R. J. A., St. Jude Children's Research Hospital, 332 North Lauderale, Memphis, TN 38101, USA

BEARD, M. E. J., Department of Haematology, St. Bartholomew's Hospital, London, E. C. 1, UK

BENNETT, J. M., Departments of Medicine and Pediatrics, The University of Rochester, School of Medicine and Dentistry, Division of Oncology and the Highland Hospital of Rochester, Rochester, NY, USA

BERGSAGEL, D. E., Princess Margaret Hospital, 500 Sherbourne Street, Toronto 5, Canada

BERNARD, J., Institut de Recherches sur les Leucémies, Hôpital Saint-Louis, 2, place du Docteur A. Fournier, 75010 Paris, France

BESSIS, M., Institut de Pathologie Cellulaire, Hôpital de Bicêtre, Université de Paris, 75 Paris, France

BOIRON, M., Institut de Recherches sur les Maladies du Sang, Hôpital Saint-Louis, 2, place de Docteur A. Fournier, 75010 Paris, France

BORELLA, L., St. Jude Children's Research Hospital, 332 North Lauderale, Memphis, TN 38101, USA

BURCHENAL, J. H., Sloan-Kettering Institute for Cancer Research, Division of Chemotherapy Research, Memorial Hospital for Cancer and Allied Diseases and Cornell University Medical College, New York, NY, USA

CARTER, S. K., National Cancer Institute, N. I. H., Bethesda, MD 20014, USA

CATTAN, A., C.R.L.C., 45 rue Coqnacq Jay, 51100 Reims, France

CLARKSON, B. D., Sloan-Kettering Institute for Cancer Research, Division of Chemotherapy Research, Memorial Hospital for Cancer and Allied Diseases and Cornell University Medical College, New York, NY, USA

COWAN, D. H., Department of Medicine, Princess Margaret Hospital and the Ontario Cancer Institute and Sunnybrook Hospital and the University of Toronto, Toronto, Canada

CUNNINGHAM, B., Sloan-Kettering Institute for Cancer Research, Division of Chemotherapy Research, Memorial Hospital for Cancer and Allied Diseases and Cornell University Medical College, New York, NY, USA

DANIEL, M. T., Institut de Recherches sur les Leucémies et les Maladies du Sang, Hôpital Saint-Louis, 2, place de Docteur A. Fournier, 75010 Paris, France

DANTCHEV, D., Institut de Cancérologie et d'Immunogénétique, Hôpital Paul-Brousse, 14—16, Avenue Paul-Vaillant-Courturier, 94800 Villejuif, France

DeVassal, F., Unité Fred-Siguier de Dévelopment Therapeutique, Institut de Cancérologie et d'Immunogénétique, Hôpital Paul-Brousse, 14—16, Avenue Paul-Vaillant-Couturier, 94800 Villejuif, France

Dowling, M. D., Sloan-Kettering Institute for Cancer Research, Division of Chemotherapy Research, Memorial Hospital for Cancer and Allied Diseases and Cornell University Medical College, New York, NY, USA

Flandrin, G., Institut de Recherches sur les Leucémies et les Maladies du Sang, Hôpital Saint-Louis, 2, place du Docteur A. Fournier, 75010 Paris, France

Frei, III, E., Texas Medical Center, Anderson Hospital, Houston, TX 77025, USA

Gavosto, F., Division of Hematology, General Medical Clinic, University of Turin, Turin, Italy

Gee, T. S., Sloan-Kettering Institute for Cancer Research, Division of Chemotherapy Research, Memorial Hospital for Cancer and Allied Diseases and Cornell University Medical College, New York, NY, USA

Gemon, M.-F., Institut de Recherches sur les Maladies du Sang, Hôpital Saint-Louis, 2, place du Docteur A. Fournier, 75010 Paris, France

Glidewell, O., Department of Medicine, Jewish Hospital Brooklyn and State University of New York, Downstate Medical Center, Brooklyn, NY 11239, USA

Green, A. A., St. Jude Children's Research Hospital, 332 North Lauderale, Memphis, TN 38101, USA

Hacker, B., American Cancer Society Research Professor RP-42, Division of Oncology, University of Rochester, Medical Center, Rochester, NY, USA

Haghbin, M., Sloan-Kettering Institute for Cancer Research, Division of Chemotherapy Research, Memorial Hospital for Cancer and Allied Diseases and Cornell University Medical College, New York, NY, USA

Hall, T. C., American Cancer Society Research Professor RP-42, Division of Oncology, University of Rochester, Medical Center, Rochester, NY, USA

Hart, J. S., Texas Medical Center, Anderson Hospital, Houston, TX 77025, USA

Hayat, M., Unité Fred-Siguier de Dévelopment Therapeutique, Institut de Cancérologie et d'Immunogénétique, Hôpital Paul-Brousse, 14—16, Avenue Paul-Vaillant-Couturier, 94800 Villejuif, France

Izrael, V., Institut de Recherches sur les Maladies du Sang, Hôpital Saint-Louis, 2, place du Docteur A. Fournier, 75010 Paris, France

Jacquillat, Cl., Institute de Recherches sur les Leucémies, Hôpital Saint-Louis, 2, place de Docteur A. Fournier, 75010 Paris, France

Jasmin, C., Service d'Hêmatologie de l'Institut Gustave-Roussy, Hôpital Paul-Brousse, 14—16 Avenue Paul-Vaillant-Couturier, 94800 Villejuif, France

Karon, M., Division of Hematology, Department of Pediatrics, Children's Hospital of Los Angeles and the USC School of Medicine, Los Angeles, CA 90027, USA

Kessel, D., American Cancer Society Research Professor RP-42 Division of Oncology, University of Rochester, Medical Center, Rochester, NY, USA

Klemperer, M. R., Departments of Medicine and Pediatrics, The University of Rochester, School of Medicine and Dentistry, Division of Oncology and the Highland Hospital of Rochester, Rochester, NY, USA

Lafleur, M., Service d'Hématologie de l'Institut Gustave Roussy, 16 bis Avenue Paul-Vaillant-Couturier, 94800 Villejuif, France.

LEE, S. L., Department of Medicine, Jewish Hospital Brooklyn and State University of New York, Downstate Medical Center, Brooklyn, NY 11239, USA

LÖFFLER, H., Medizinische Kliniken und Polikliniken der Justus-Liebig Universität, 6300 Gießen, Germany

MATHÉ, G., Institut de Cancérologie et d'Immunogénétique, Hôpital Paul Brousse, 14—16 Avenue Paul-Vaillant-Couturier, 94800 Villejuif, France

MCCULLOCH, E. A., Department of Medicine, Princess Margaret Hospital and the Ontario Cancer Institute and Sunnybrook Hospital and the University of Toronto, Toronto, Canada

MESSNER, H. A., Department of Medicine, Princess Margaret Hospital and the Ontario Cancer Institute and Sunnybrook Hospital and the University of Toronto, Toronto, Canada

NAHAS, A., American Cancer Society Research Professor RP-42 Division of Oncology, University of Rochester, Medical Center, Rochester, NY, USA

PAINTRAND, M., Institut de Cancérologie et d'Immunogénétique, Hôpital Paul-Brousse, 14—16 Avenue Paul-Vaillant-Couturier, 94800 Villejuif, France

PERRY, S., National Cancer Institute, N.I.H., Bethesda, MD 20014, USA

PIKE, M. C., DHSS Cancer Epidemiology and Clinical Trials Unit, Department of the Regius, Professor of Medicine, Oxford University, 9 Keble Road, Oxford, England

PINKEL, D., St. Jude Children's Research Hospital, 332 North Lauderale Memphis, TN 38101, USA

POUILLART, P., Institut de Cancérologie et d'Immunogénétique, Hôpital Paul-Brousse, 14—16 Avenue Paul Vaillant-Couturier, 94800 Villejuif, France

RAPPAPORT, H., Department of Pathology, The School of Medicine of the University of Chicago, Chicago, IL., USA

ROSENFELD, C., Service d'Hématologie de l'Institut Gustave-Roussy, Hôpital Paul-Brousse, 14—16 Paul-Vaillant-Couturier, 94800 Villejuif, France

SCHNEIDER, M., C.A.C., 36 Avenue de la Voie Romaine, 06000 Nice, France

SCHWARZENBERG, L., Unité Fred-Siguieur de Dévelopment Therapeutique, Institut de Cancérologie et d'Immunogénétique, Hôpital Paul-Brousse, 14—16 Avenue Paul-Vaillant-Couturier, 94800 Villejuif, France

SEGEL, G. B., Departments of Medicine and Pediatrics, The University of Rochester, School of Medicine and Dentistry, Division of Oncology and the Highland Hospital of Rochester, Rochester, NY, USA

SENN, J. S., Department of Medicine, Princess Margaret Hospital and the Ontario Cancer Institute and Sunnybrook Hospital and the University of Toronto, Toronto, Canada

SIMONE, J. V., St. Jude Children's Research Hospital, 332 North Lauderale, Memphis, TN 38101, USA

STERESCO, M., Service d'Hématologie de l'Institut Gustave Roussy, 14—16 Avenue Paul-Vaillant-Couturier, 98400 Villejuif, France

TAN, C. T. C., Sloan-Kettering Institute for Cancer Research, Division of Chemotherapy Research, Memorial Hospital for Cancer and Allied Diseases and Cornell University Medical College, New York, NY, USA

WEIL, M., Institute de Recherches sur les Leucemies, Hôpital Saint-Louis, 2, place de Docteur A. Fournier, 75010 Paris, France

WEINER, R., Division of Medical Oncology Harvard University Medical School Boston, MA., USA

General Introduction

Scientific and Ethical Discipline in Clinical Trials on Acute Leukemia

G. MATHÉ

Institut de Cancérologie et d'Immunogénétique *, Hôpital Paul-Brousse **, Villejuif/France

Clinical research is still in an evolutionary stage. Although scientific technology was readily accepted and applied, scientific methodology has been accepted much more slowly and is very rarely properly applied. There are three reasons why this is so.

First, medical ethics frequently limits the applicability of clinical research, for doctors have to be more than scientists. They must also remain moral philosophers, as they were before medicine became a science.

Second, the heterogeneity of the material on which clinical researchers work in studying human diseases makes the application of scientific methodology difficult.

Third, researchers must publish. This means that they must obtain publishable results, and too often this means results in accordance with established concepts, easily accepted by the editors of established journals, which are read by the establishment.

It is the privilege of too many people to be able to accept "truth" and recipes from other people and confirm their truth and results. It is the mission of a very few others to accept nothing as "truth" and to consider no recipe ideal, either in concept or detail.

This meeting has been organized in order to assemble people of this last type. We are here neither to find a compromised truth nor to write a recipe from the sum or average of all the recipes. We are here, rather, to allow a confrontation of scientific methods and ethical rules in order to elevate both, and to allow a confrontation of the results of different techniques of treatment in order to improve them.

The acute leukemias belong to a group of diseases the prognosis of which is improving for some varieties but not for others. We must discuss why this is so and try to speak the same language. Several types of therapeutical approaches are available and have been applied. They are chemotherapy, active immunotherapy, adoptive immunotherapy, and bone marrow replacement. All of these have made great advances. The indications for their use, however, should no longer depend upon the geographic location of the patient or of this physician but on the variety of his disease. We have shown that there are patients with acute lymphoid leukemia whose five-year life expectancy with active immunotherapy is more than 90% and incidence of death

---

* INSERM et Association Claude-Bernard.

** 14—16, av. Paul-Vaillant Couturier.

0%. In other varieties, the survival expectancy with active immunotherapy at five years is almost nil. We have to learn about the effects of chemotherapy on these different varieties.

A strictly controlled scientific trial conducted on acute myeloid leukemia (AML) by the EORTC Leukemia Group has indicated a very low percentage of complete remissions. Hence, the International Cooperative Group on Bone Marrow transplantation is planning to return to adoptive immunotherapy and bone marrow replacement in treating this disease. This is a logical treatment, because this neoplasia seems to affect the complete hemopoietic system, and it is ethical for those whose prognosis as predicted by cytology is very poor.

This meeting is also one of a series of meetings that traditionally bring together EORTC members and their American colleagues. I would like to welcome all the participants and thank the institutions which contributed to its organization, especially the American NCI, Euratom, EORTC, and the French CNRS and INSERM.

First Session
Nomenclature and Classification

Introduction to Nomenclature and Classification of Acute Leukemias

S. Perry

National Cancer Institute, N.I.H., Bethesda, MD/USA

The nomenclature and classification of acute leukemia has been a source of concern and controversy since the earliest clinical description of leukemia nearly 150 years ago. In 1827, Velpeau (cited by Dameshek and Gunz, 1964) described a 63-year-old patient, a florist and seller of lemonade, "who had abandoned himself to the abuse of spirituous liquor and of women without, however, becoming syphilitic", who presented with an enlarged abdomen, fever and weakness. He died promptly and at autopsy, in addition to hepatosplenomegaly, the blood was thick "like gruel ... resembling in consistency and color the yeast of red wine ... One might have asked if it were not rather laudable pus ... than blood." Donné in Paris was the first to examine the blood of such a patient microscopically and found more than half of it to consist of "mucous globules" which could not be distinguished from pus corpuscles. Since the relation between the red corpuscles and the white corpuscles was the reverse of normal, Virchow used the term "white blood" to describe the condition. In 1847, he introduced the name "leukemia" and published a series of papers on the nature of the disease which he classified into two forms, "splenic" associated with splenomegaly and "lymphatic" characterized by lymph node enlargement and the presence of white corpuscles in the blood resembling those in the lymph nodes.

By 1857, the two types of chronic leukemia and the acute variety had been recognized (Dameshek and Gunz [1]; Wintrobe [7]), although no one had clearly designated cases with a rapidly fatal course until Ebstein's report in 1889. However, morphologic methods were crude and for years it was believed that acute leukemia was only lymphocytic in nature.

The last quarter of the 19th century was a period of rapid progress in cytologic techniques and included Ehrlich's discovery of staining methods which made it possible for the first time to study cellular details and to describe characteristic morphologic features associated with various types of leukemia. Ehrlich introduced differential staining methods and in 1891 published a classic monograph which stimulated research and observations in leukemias. He described the specific granules of leukocytes and developed the classification of white blood cells into neutrophils, basophils and eosinophils. His studies also led to a division of leukemia into two major types, the "spleno-myelogenous" type consisting of large numbers of neutrophils and mononuclear cells containing specific granules and the "lymphocytic" type with many mononuclear leukocytes not containing granules. The acute terminal phase of chronic myelocytic leukemia was recognized but was considered to be a transformation from myelocytic to lymphocytic leukemia.

However, with Naegeli's description of the myeloblast in 1900 much of the confusion was clarified. It became apparent that there were at least two forms of acute leukemia, myelocytic and lymphocytic. The concept of transformation was largely abandoned and the occurrence of different phases of leukemia with varying proportions of mature and immature cells was recognized. The myeloblast was established as the early precursor of the myeloid series in both normal and leukemic marrows and its distinction from immature cells of the lymphocytic series was accepted (Hayhoe [4]).

The introduction of the peroxidase stain in 1916 and development of other cytologic and cytochemical techniques in the next two decades did not unfortunately resolve all the problems and controversy about nomenclature and classification. The Romanowsky stains remained the most important technique for cytologic discrimination amongst the leukemic cells, but careful attention was given to precise descriptions of every cellular structure and characteristic which might be of value for cell identification. These included most of the features currently in use such as Auer rods, nucleoli, characteristics of nuclear chromatin, etc.

Eventually, the two major divisions of the acute leukemias, lymphocytic and myeloid, were divided further based on the predominant cell type and it was recognized that there were myeloblastic forms of acute leukemia, promyelocytic, monomyelocytic, monoblastic, and promonocytic types and forms in which early erythroid and megakaryocytic cells were prominent in the blood and bone marrow. Additional categories and designations have also been proposed based on some specific characteristic of the cell type observed such as "microlymphoblasts", "macrolymphoblasts", etc. (Mathé *et al.*, 1971) or on the variety of cells such as erythremic myelosis (Hayhoe, Quaglino, and Doll [3]). However, most of these designations have not been widely employed.

In any case, with the recognition of the acute leukemias in the early 1900's, the predominant emphasis on morphologic hematology came to an end and in subsequent decades the major attention in research to distinguish the leukemias was given to other approaches—clinical, cytochemical, functional, cytogenetic, biochemical, ultra-structural, kinetic, immunologic, etc. These will be discussed during the course of this workshop.

Recent developments in automated image-processing, however, may ultimately have an important impact on the classification of leukemias (Lipkin [5]). There are a number of such efforts in the United States and Europe which should come to fruition in the near future. Classification of white blood cells has always depended on examination of Romanowsky stained marrow and blood smears by a morphologist of one kind or another. Categorization of cells has been based on parameters expressible largely in qualitative terms such as "finely stippled", "vacuolated", "ground glass", "coarse", etc. In automated image-processing, analytical techniques will be used to quantify cells as to density, texture, shape and other fine characteristics.

The inadequacy of classifying acute leukemias on the basis of current cytological staining techniques remains obvious. Studies such as the one described by Hayhoe *et al.* (Hayhoe, Quaglino, and Doll [3]), have repeatedly demonstrated that hematologists and pathologists frequently do not agree about cytologic classification, particularly in acute leukemia. Worse still, when an individual reviewer re-examines a slide, his diagnosis often differs from his original opinion.

The attempts to classify the leukemias I have just described could have been considered academic were it not for the observations by Farber in 1948 (FARBER *et al.* [2]) that folic acid antagonists could be used successfully in the treatment of one type of acute leukemia, acute lymphoblastic leukemia in children, and that other forms were relatively resistant. Subsequent years have reinforced the importance of accurate diagnosis in patients presenting with leukemia of any type (MATHÉ *et al.* [6]).

Finally, even from this brief discussion, it is obvious that classification based on staining characteristics and cell morphology has been intensively investigated for many decades; used by themselves, however, these features are not adequate. Morphologic characteristics as well as subcellular studies, functional behavior, biochemical characterization, cytochemical evaluation and other techniques all have to be utilized for the precise classification of the leukemias.

References

1. DAMESHEK, W., GUNZ, F.: Leukemia. 2nd Edition, p. 1. New York: Grune & Stratton 1964.
2. FARBER, S. *et al.*: Temporary remissions in acute leukemia in children produced by folic acid antagonist, 4-aminopteroy-glutamic acid (aminopterin). New Engl. J. Med. **238**, 787 (1948).
3. HAYHOE, F. G. J., QUAGLINO, D., DOLL, R.: The cytology and cytochemistry of acute leukaemias. London: Her Majesty's Stationery Office 1964.
4. HAYHOE, F. G. J.: Leukaemia research and clinical practice. p. 1. Boston: Little, Brown and Co. 1960.
5. LIPKIN, L.: Unpublished observations 1972.
6. MATHÉ, G. *et al.*: Subdivision of classical varieties of acute leukemia. Correlation with prognosis and cure expectancy. Europ. J. clin. biol. Res. **16**, 554—560 (1971).
7. WINTROBE, M. M.: Clinical hematology. 6th Ed., p. 982. Philadelphia: Lea and Febiger 1967.

Classification and Subclassification of Acute Leukemias Correlated with Clinical Expression, Therapeutic Sensitivity and Prognosis

G. Mathé, P. Pouillart, R. Weiner, M. Hayat, Marina Steresco, and Marguerite Lafleur

Institut de Cancérologie et d'Immunogénétique *, Hôpital Paul-Brousse **, Villejuif/France

Hemopoietic and lymphoid cell physiology has been progressing very rapidly, particularly since the results of the first bone marrow transplantation experiments (see [7]), thymectomy experiments [12], and bone marrow [1, 15, 16] and lymphocyte in vitro culture [13] became available. However, morphology has not kept pace with these other disciplines and has not shown any significant progress recently. Since McCullogh, one of the greatest living hematologists, has declared: "Hematology must do without the microscope", one is reluctant to propose a new morphological classification or subclassification of a "well-established" group of diseases.

Nevertheless, that is what we intend to do; and we shall do it for acute leukemias (AL), although some colleagues may believe that this is useless because, in their opinion, therapeutic success are applied to any morphologic variety or subvariety of AL.

The usefulness of the recent subclassification of Hodgkin's disease [5] encourages us to propose one for the AL, and this paper will show that, until new therapeutic measures (against AL) are introduced, such a subclassification can be very useful, especially for therapeutic indications and prognosis.

One of us (G. M.) has for the last six years been in charge of the World Health Organization (WHO) Reference Center for Nomenclature and Classification of Neoplasias of the Hemopoietic and Lymphoid Cells [11]. We have attempted to establish a classification of the malignant diseases of the hematopoietic and lymphoid tissues which would be universally acceptable, because the techniques required are simple, and reliable, because there is reproducibility of interpretation by the same microscopist and by different microscopists.

Through classifying the cells in bone marrow smears stained by the May-Grunwald-Giemsa method prior to initiation of therapy according to cell lines and degree of differentiation, we came to the following conclusions (Table 1). Three varieties can be easily recognized: 1. *"acute lymphoid leukemia"* (ALL), 2. *"acute myeloid leuke-*

---

* INSERM et Association Claude-Bernard.

** 14—16, av. Paul-Vaillant Couturier.

Table 1. The characters of the leukemic cells which help to classify them according to the three lines and the four varietes of Acute Leukemia (AL) according to the lines

	Lymphoid	Myeloid	Monocytoid
Cytoplasm	No azurophilic granules	Delicate azurophilic granules At times, Auer bodies	Possible very delicate azurophilic granules
Nucleus	One or no nucleolus visible	Several nucleoli	Distorted Several nucleoli
Nucleo-cytoplasmic ratio	High	Average	Low
Leukemia	Acute Lymphoid (ALL)	Acute Myeloid (AML) Acute Myelo-Monocytoid (MMoAL)	Acute Monocytoid (MocAL)

mia" (AML) and 3. "*acute monocytoid leukemia*" (AMoL). In addition, there is an acute leukemia where either the cells look as much monocytoid as myeloid, or there is a mixture of myeloid and monocytoid elements; this variety has been called "*acute myelomonocytoid leukemia*" (MMoAL). Table 2 indicates that, within each main group (lymphoid, myeloid, and monocytoid), three subvarieties can be distinguished: (1) "*blastic*" and (2) "*procytic*" easily, and (3) "*problastic*" with relatively more difficulty. Moreover, in ALL we had to separate two types for the "blastic" varieties according to the diameter of the cells (Table 2), namely "*macrolymphoblastic*" and "*microlymphoblastic*". In other words, we proposed a subclassification of ALL into four varieties: "*prolymphoblastic*" AL (PLbAL), "*macrolymphoblastic*" AL (MLbAL), "*microlymphoblastic*" AL (mLbAL) and "*prolymphocytic*" AL (PLcAL). Fig. 1 (plate) shows these four subvarieties of ALL, the three subvarieties of AML, "*promyeloblastic*" AL (PMbAL), "*myeloblastic*" AL (MbAL) and "*promyelocytic*" AL (PMcAL), and the three subvarieties of AMoL, "*promonoblastic*" (PMobAL), "*monoblastic*" (MobAL) and "*promonocytic*" (PMocAL). It shows also two examples of the *myelomonocytoid* type (MMoAL).

Table 2. The names given by convention to the cells according to their degree of differentiation and to the leukemias according to the cells which predominate

	Lymphoid	Myeloid	Monocytoid
Typical blasts	Macrolymphoblasts [a] (MLbAL) Microlymphoblasts [b] (mLbAL)	Myeloblasts (MbAL)	Monoblasts (MobAL)
Less differentiated	Prolymphoblasts (PLbAL)	Promyeloblasts (PMbAL)	Promonoblasts (PMobAL)
More differentiated	Prolymphocytes (PLcAL)	Promyelocytes (PMcAL)	Promonocytes (PMocAL)

[a] Diameter $\geqq 11\ \mu$. [b] Diameter $\leqq 11\ \mu$.

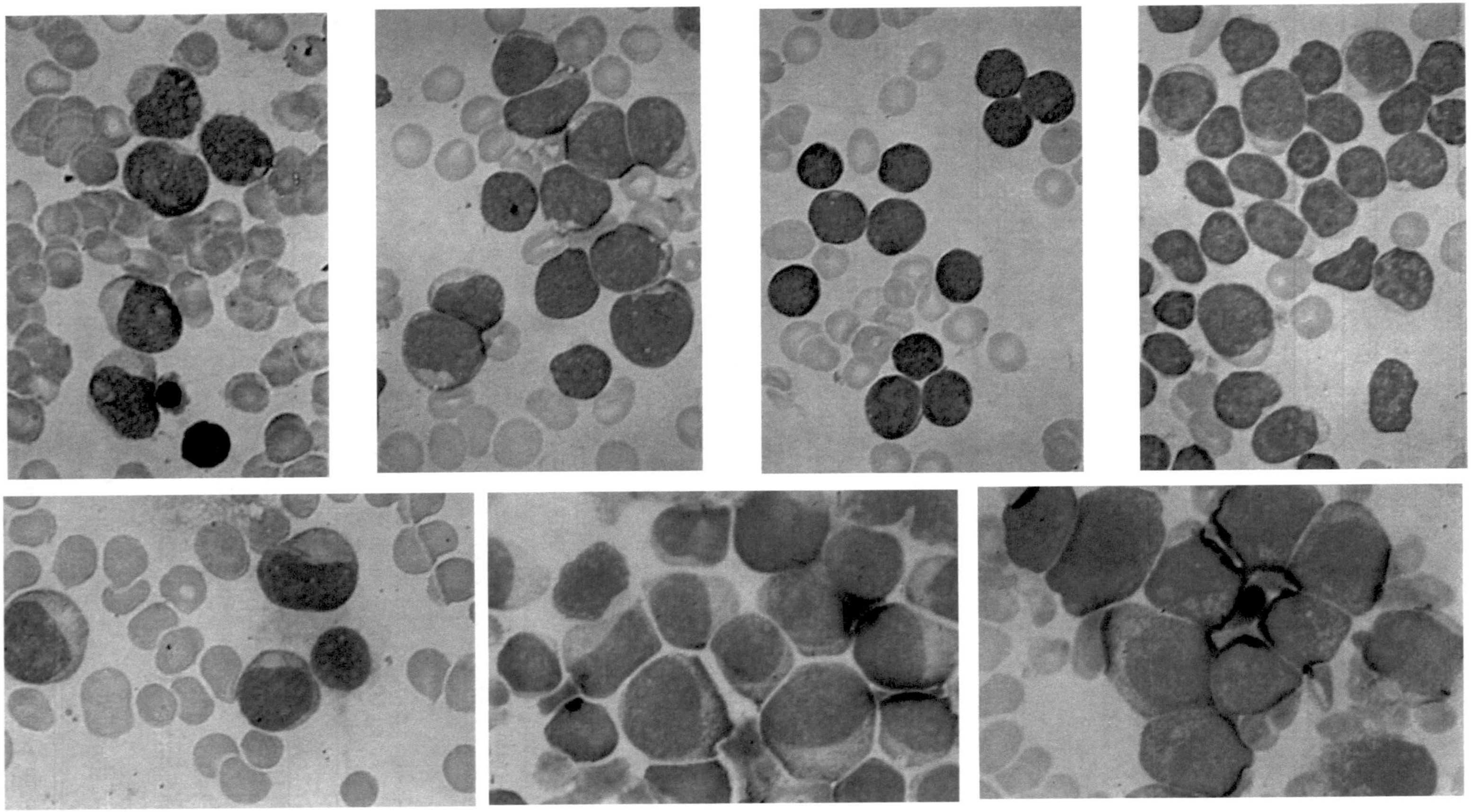

Fig. 1 a—g (Plate 1)

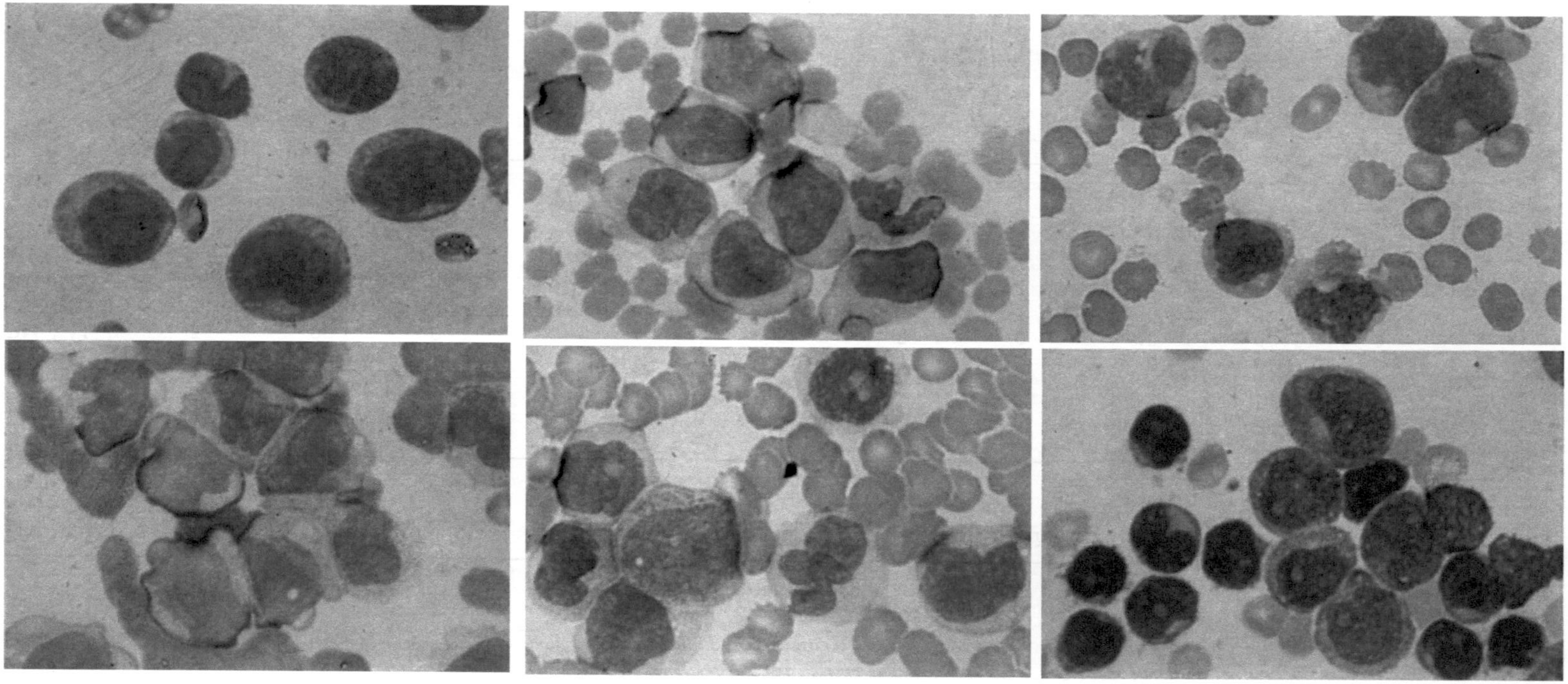

Fig. 1 h—n (Plate 2)

Fig. 1 a—n. (Plate 1+2) The different subvarieties of acute leukemias. a Acute lymphoid leukemia prolymphoblastic (PLbAL), b acute lymphoid leukemia macrolymphoblastic (MlbAL), c acute lymphoid leukemia microlymphoblastic (mLbAL), d acute lymphoid leukemia prolymphocytic (PLcAL), e acute myeloid leukemia promyeloblastic (PMbAL), f acute myeloid leukemia myeloblastic (MbAL), g acute myeloid leukemia promyelocytic (PMcAL), h acute monocytoid leukemia promonoblastic (PMobAL), i acute monocytoid leukemia monoblastic (MobAL), k acute monocytoid leukemia promonocytic (PMocAL), l and m acute myelomonocytoid leukemia (AMMOL), n acute myeloid leukemia rich in lymphoblast-like cells

Table 3. Index of Changing (IC) in the double blind evaluation by the same observor

$$IC = \frac{\text{Number of changes}}{\begin{matrix}\text{Number of cases}\\ \text{of one variety}\end{matrix} + \begin{matrix}\text{Number of cases}\\ \text{of the other variety}\end{matrix}} \quad (\%)$$

GM versus GM	PLbAL	MLbAL	mLbAL	PLcAL	PMobAL	MobAL	PMocAL	MMoAL	PMbAL	TMbAL	PMcAL
PLbAL		22	0	0	5	0	0	0	0	0	0
MLbAL	22		3	3	0	0	0	0	0	0	0
mLbAL	0	3		14	0	0	0	0	0	0	0
PLcAL	0	3	14		0	0	0	0	0	0	0
PMobAL	5	0	0	0		5	0	0	18	0	0
MobAL	0	0	0	0	5		0	5	0	0	0
PMocAL	0	0	0	0	0	0		7	0	0	0
MMoAL	0	0	0	0	0	5	7		3	2	0
PMbAL	0	0	0	0	18	0	0	3		6	0
TMbAL	0	0	0	0	0	0	0	2	6		0
PMcAL	0	0	0	0	0	0	0	0	0	0	

Table 4. Index of Changing (IC) in the double blind evaluation by two observors

$$IC = \frac{\text{Number of changes}}{\text{Number of cases of one variety} + \text{Number of cases of the other variety}} (\%)$$

GM versus S	PLbAL	MLbAL	mLbAL	PLcAL	PMobAL	MobAL	PMocAL	MMoAL	PMbAL	TMbAL	PMcAL
PLbAL		10	0	0	0	0	0	0	0	0	0
MLbAL	10		6	4	0	0	0	0	0	0	0
mLbAL	0	6		14	0	0	0	0	0	0	0
PLcAL	0	4	14		0	0	0	0	0	0	0
PMobAL	0	0	0	0		12.5	0	4	7	3	0
MobAL	0	0	0	0	12.5		0	4	0	0	0
PMocAL	0	0	0	0	0	0		0	0	0	0
MMoAL	0	0	0	0	4	4	0		4	4	0
PMbAL	0	0	0	0	7	0	0	4		10	0
TMbAL	0	0	0	0	3	0	0	4	10		0
PMcAL	0	0	0	0	0	0	0	0	0	0	

That the reproducibility is satisfactory was demonstrated by two tests conducted in a double blind fashion (one observer, a physician GM, versus himself, and one observer versus another observer, a technician) (Tables 3 and 4). It can be seen that the main difficulty concerns the distinction between the PLbAL and the MLbAL subvarieties.

The correlations between the features of the cells used for this routine classification and those of (a) cytochemistry data, (b) electron microscopy aspects, (c) behavior in in-vitro cultures on agar, (d) behavior in cultures in suspension, (e) kinetic behavior, and (f) their antigenic and immunogenic characteristics, are under study in cooperation with Hayhoe, Paintrand [14], Pouillart [17], Belpomme and Doré respectively (Table 5).

Table 5. Expected help in classification of acute leukemias

From	For
Cytochemistry	?
Electron microscopy	MMoAL The four varieties of ALL
Culture on Agar	Distinction between the less differentiated AML and ALL
in suspension	?
Antigenic and immunogenic characteristics	Distinction between ALL and AML

In this paper, we shall merely point out that there is some correlation between this classification and therapeutic sensitivity on the one hand, and prognosis on the other. We shall choose three examples to illustrate them.

1. The importance of *distinguishing MMoAL from AML* is shown by the fact that the myeloid leukemic cells may disappear after administration of cytosine arabinoside (CAR), or a combination of CAR with thioguanine (THG), or CAR with daunorubicine (DRB), while the monocytoid cells may persist [4]. We were able to "complete" the remission in several patients by administering 4-demethyl-epipodophyllotoxin B.D. ethenylidene or EPE or VP16213 (Fig. 2), which is the compound to which monocytoid leukemic cells are the most sensitive [3, 8]. Hence we suggest that a diagnosis of MMoAL is an indication for treatment with a combination of CAR and VP16213. VP16213 has had no effect in pure AML and CAR is ineffective in pure AMoL.

2. The second example concerns the results obtained by the EORTC "Leukaemia and Hematosarcoma" Group in a controlled trial of AML and MMoAL treatment by CAR or CAR + THG or CAR + DRB. The acceptance of a patient into the trial and the designation of the therapeutic result as a "complete remission" (CR) depended on a double blind examination of (a) the smear at the time of the initial diagnosis, (b) a second smear at the time of remission. One can see from Table 6 that the incidence of CR may be a little higher in the myeloblastic type than in the promyelocytic or the promyeloblastic variety. But the difference is not yet significant. More interesting is the following fact: we have distinguished in this double blind examination

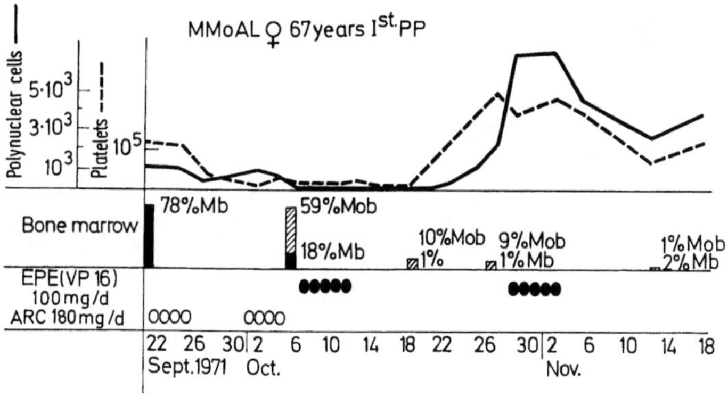

Fig. 2. Acute myelomonocytoid leukemias: the myeloblasts were much reduced after CAR course while the monoblasts increased. The latter disappeared after a VP16 213 course

Table 6. Incidence of "complete" remissions in AML according to the cytological subvariety. (EORTC "Leukemia and Hematosarcoma" Group) (Trial AML_1, 1970—1971, CAR vs CAR+THG vs CAR+DRB)

	Number of cases	Complete remissions		
Promyeloblastic	59	5	8%	NS
Myeloblastic	45	10	22%	
Promyelocytic	11	1	10%	
Myelo-monocytoid	25	4	16%	
AML subvarieties (without "Lymphoblast-like" cells)	141	20	14%	S ($p < 0.01$)
AML subvarieties (with many "Lymphoblast-like" cells)	23	9	39%	

of the AML or the MMoAL *those smears which contain only typical granulocytic or monocytoid cells* and *those which show at the same time many cells presenting all the features of the cells which characterize ALL* (see Fig. 1, plate): we have called these cells *"lymphoblast-like" cells* and called these leukemias *"AML with many lymphoblast-like cells"*. Table 7 shows that the incidence of CR is significantly higher in this group of AML than in those not presenting these features, and Fig. 3 shows that patients in this group have a longer survival time, while Fig. 4. demonstrates that those who have a CR remain in this condition for longer.

The question is now whether these myeloid leukemias, which we have called "myeloid leukemia with many lymphoblast-like cells" are: 1. myeloid leukemia with many cells in Go or long G_1, 2. mixed myelolymphoid leukemias, or 3. lymphoid leukemias with granulocytic reactions. This problem is currently under study. The

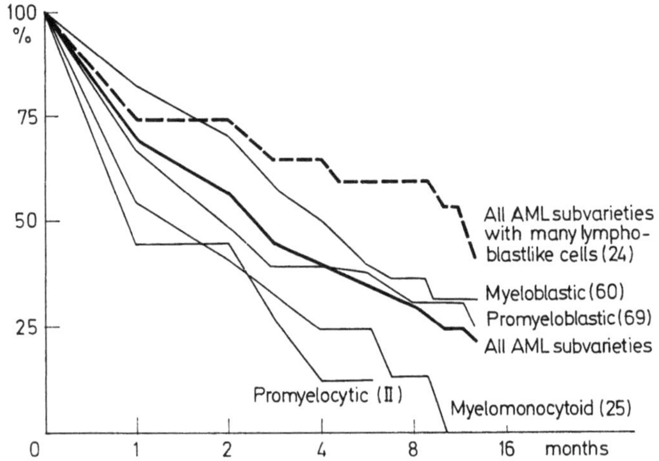

Fig. 3. Actuarial curve of cumulative survival of all AML patients submitted to trial ALM[1] (1970—1971) (CAR or CAR+THG or CAR+DRB) (EORTC "Leukemia and Hematosarcoma group), according to the different cytological varieties

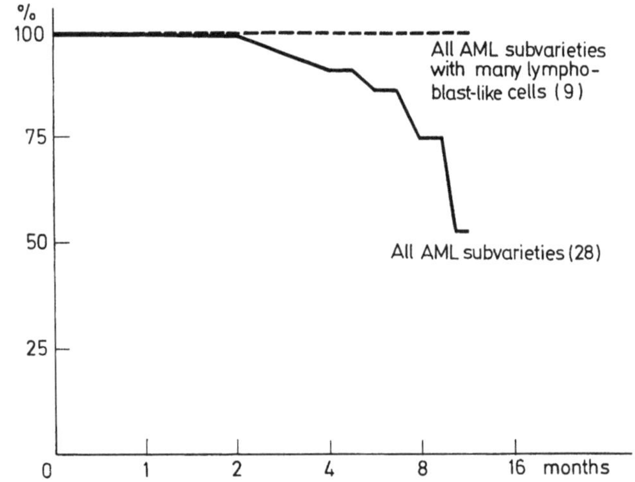

Fig. 4. Actuarial curves of cumulative duration of "complete" remissions of AML patients submitted to trial AML[1] (1970—1971) (CAR or CAR+THG or CAR+DRB) (EORTC "Leukemia and Hematosarcoma" group), according to the abundant presence of "lymphoblast-like" cells on the first smear

most important knowledge we have gained from this special designation is that these forms have a better prognosis and therefore should be deleted from risk-bearing therapeutic protocols which may not be unreasonable in AML patients.

3. The most interesting observation concerns the correlation between the *subclassification of ALL* on the one hand, and symptomatology, therapeutic sensitivity

and prognosis on the other hand. We shall consider in this report 100 patients whose bone marrow smears obtained prior to any therapy we reviewed in a recent work [10]. All these patients were treated according to a protocol comprising three phases: chemotherapy to induce remission; pre-immunotherapy cell-reducing complementary systemic chemotherapy and chemoradiotherapy of the central nervous system (CNS); and finally active immunotherapy [6, 9] (Fig. 5).

The relative incidence of the four varieties is given in Fig. 6 for all patients, and for patients under 15 years of age. The relative incidence in males and females is also indicated.

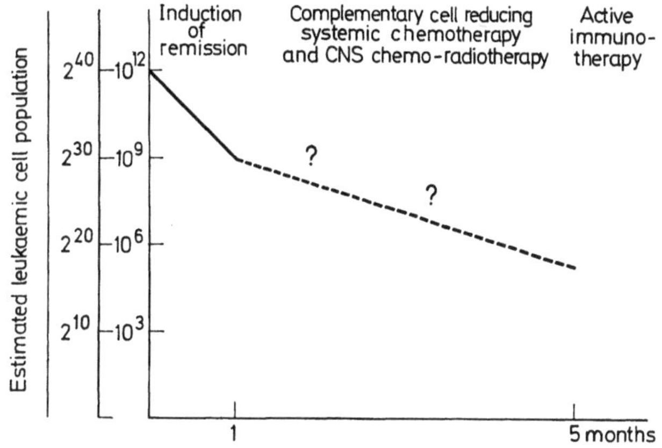

Fig. 5. Principle of the treatment protocols of ALL

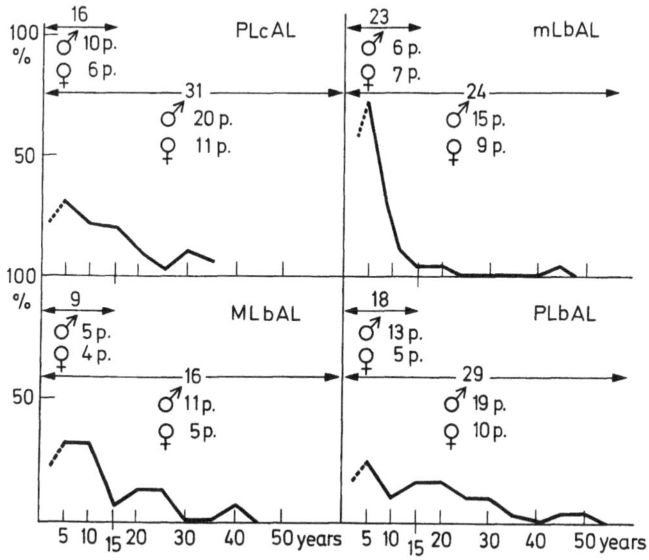

Fig. 6. Relative incidence of the four varieties of ALL for all patients and patients under 15 years of age. Relative incidence in males and females. Incidence according to age

Tables 7 and 8 show the relative incidence of splenomegaly, lymph-node enlargement, high leukemic cell levels in peripheral blood, and meningeal localization at the time of diagnosis and of meningeal and testicular localizations in relapses. We observed (a) that splenomegaly, lymph-node enlargement, and high numbers of leukemic cells in the peripheral blood are relatively more frequent in the "microlymphoblastic" and "prolymphocytic" varieties; (b) that testicular and meningeal localizations in relapse are more frequent in the "prolymphocytic" variety; and (c) that meningeal localization at the time of diagnosis is more frequent in the "prolymphoblastic" type.

More useful is the observation concerning the duration of the first apparently complete remission (CR) under immunotherapy and the total survival times for all patients, with or without relapse.

Fig. 7 shows that the actuarial curve of the first CR is, as can be seen on the left for the subjects of all ages, very different from one cytological variety to another.

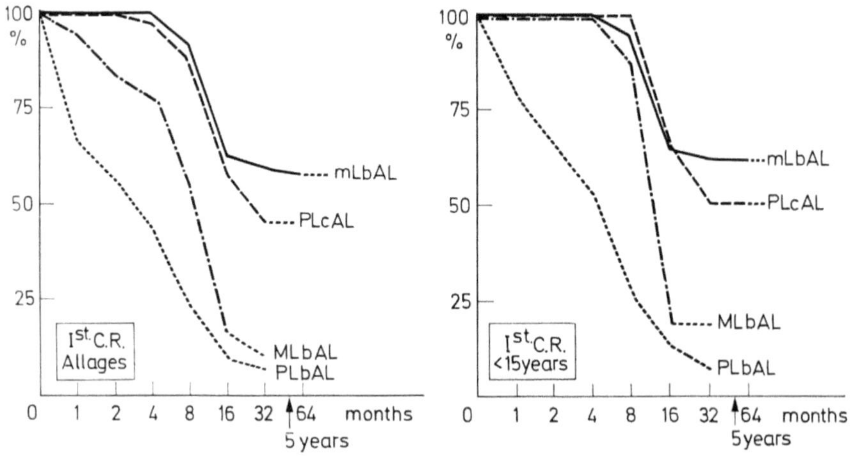

Fig. 7. Comparative cumulative total duration of first remission of the patients according to the different cytological varieties of ALL (all ages) (actuarial curves). Comparative cumulative total duration of first remission of the patients according to the different cytological varieties of ALL (patients younger than 15 years) (actuarial curves). Note that time scale is geometric

While the slopes of the curves of the PLbAL and the MLbAL varieties fall steeply to a very low percentage of remission at 16 months, those of the mLbAL and the PLcAL varieties are interrupted between 16 and 32 months by a plateau which at five years persists in about 50% of the patients. This plateau is a little higher for the mLbAL type than for the PLc one. This plateau seems short because of the necessary geometric representation of the time scale but it would appear very long with an arithmetic one. It is usually considered as the statistical expression of "cure expectancy".

On the right of Fig. 7 this plateau can be seen to be a little higher in patients below 15 years of age (65% for the mLbAL type) than for the total population of all ages.

Table 7. Some clinical manifestation according to the cellular variety (all ages)

	S+ [a]	S−	A+ [a]	A−	Blood leukemic cells [a]			Meningitis				Testis (relapses)	
					> 25,000	5,000 to 25,000	< 5,000	1st PP		Relapses			
								M+	M−	M+	M−	T+	T−
PLbAL	7/20	13/20	5/20	15/20	0/20	2/20	18/20	8/29	21/29	8/29	21/29	1/19	18/19
MLbAL	2/14	12/14	0/14	14/14	0/14	1/14	13/14	3/16	13/16	2/16	14/16	0/11	11/11
mLbAL	10/16	6/16	6/16	10/16	2/16	6/16	8/16	2/24	22/24	1/24	23/24	2/15	13/15
PLcAL	9/14	5/14	9/14	5/14	4/14	5/14	5/14	3/31	28/31	7/31	24/31	5/20	15/20

[a] Manifestations observed in the hospital before the first treatment.
PP = perceptible phase; S = splenomegaly; A = adenomegaly; M = meningeal localization; T = testis localization.

Table 8. Some clinical manifestations according to the cellular variety (< 15 years)

	S+ [a]	S−	A+ [a]	A−	Blood leukemic cells [a]			Meningitis				Testis (relapses)	
					> 25,000	5,000 to 25,000	< 5,000	1st PP		Relapses			
								M+	M−	M+	M−	T+	T−
PLbAL	5/13	8/13	3/13	10/13	0	1/13	12/13	6/18	12/18	3/18	15/18	1/19	18/19
MLbAL	1/9	8/9	0	9/9	0	1/9	8/9	2/9	7/9	1/9	8/9	0/9	9/9
mLbA	10/15	5/15	5/15	10/15	2/15	6/15	7/15	2/23	21/23	1/23	22/23	2/15	13/15
PLcAL	5/8	3/8	4/8	4/8	3/8	2/8	3/8	1/16	15/16	4/16	12/16	5/11	6/11

[a] Manifestations observed in the hospital before the first treatment.
PP = perceptible phase; S = splenomegaly; A = adenomegaly; M = meningeal localization; T = testis localization.

Fig. 8 shows the actuarial survival curves on the left for patients of all ages, and on the right for patients under 15 years. Two observations can be made: 1. There is a plateau for about 50% of the patients, not only for the two preceding varieties, PLcAL and mLbAL, but for another one, the MLbAL type: this difference between duration of the first CR under immunotherapy and length of actuarial survival suggests that, while the mLbAL and the PLcAL types are sensitive to immunotherapy, the MLbAL type is not, but is sensitive to chemotherapy. In fact, when a patient relapses under immunotherapy, he is again submitted to chemotherapy for remission induction, followed by pre-immunotherapy chemotherapy, and finally immunotherapy.

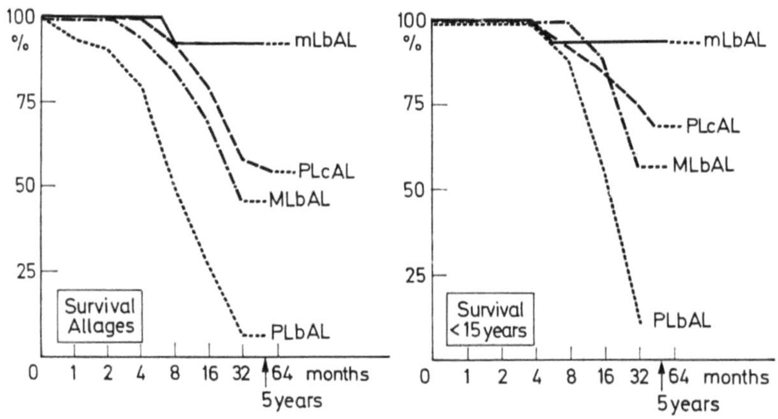

Fig. 8. Comparative cumulative survival of the ALL patients according to the cytological variety (all ages) (actuarial curves). Comparative cumulative survival of the ALL patients according to the cytological varieties (patients younger than 15 years) (actuarial curves). Note that time scale is geometrical

This observation is very important for determining the therapeutic protocols; since 1964 we have been treating all our ALL patients (except for one trial) with remission-induction chemotherapy, then complementary cell-reducing chemoradiotherapy then active immunotherapy. Except for one trial, chemotherapy has been moderate in intensity and duration [10]. It has been responsible for no therapeutic deaths. Other groups have been submitting patients to intensive and/or very long so called "maintenance chemotherapy". The accidents and deaths attributable to such treatment are not rare, being as high as 16% in some reports [18] and more in others (GLIDEWELL, pers. comm.; MIESCHER, pers. comm.).

It therefore seems that the choice between (a) protocols comprising moderate chemotherapy followed by immunotherapy, and (b) protocols comprising intensive and/or long-term chemotherapy, can be determined by the cytological type: while it is indicated to submit the mLbAL and PLcAL types to moderate chemotherapy followed by immunotherapy, it does not seem unreasonable to take some risks with a more intensive and longer chemotherapy for the other types, especially the MLbAL variety.

2. The other observation extracted from those curves is the prognostic value of this apparently sophisticated but technically simple classification. As indicated by the figure, if we see mainly microlymphoblasts on the first bone marrow smear, we can say to the family of a patient that there is about a 90% chance that the patient will be alive in five years; this variety is thus one of the prognostically most favorable neoplastic diseases with respect to five-year survival.

We know from BURCHENAL's study [2] that the exceptional long-term survivors after a conventional treatment can still relapse after five years. Though we have as yet not had any relapse after this time, it is still too early to know whether immunotherapy will avoid such very late relapses and, at the present time, the plateau phenomenon can be interpreted only as an expression of "cure expectancy".

References

1. BRADLEY, T. R., METCALF, D.: The growth of mouse bone marrow cells in vitro. Aust. J. exp. biol. med. Sci. **44**, 287 (1966).
2. BURCHENAL, J. H.: Long-term survivors in acute leukemia. p. 167. In: Advances in the treatment of acute (blastic) leukemias. 1 vol., Heidelberg: Springer 1970.
3. E.O.R.T.C.: Clinical screening of 4-demethyl-epipodophyllotoxin B.D. thenylidene coside (VP 16) in acute leukemias, hematosarcomas and solid tumors. Brit. Med. J. **3**, 199 (1973).
4. E.O.R.T.C: Leukaemia and Hematosarcoma Coop. Group. A controlled trial in acute myeloid leukaemia, comparing CAR, CAR combined with THG and CAR combined with DRB. Absence of difference. Biomedicine **18**, 192 (1973).
5. LUKES, R. J., CRAVER, L., HALL, T., RAPPAPORT, H., RUBIN, P.: Report on nomenclature Committee. Cancer Res. **26** (part 1), 1311 (1966).
6. MATHÉ, G.: Active immunotherapy. Advanc. Cancer Res. **14**, 1 (1971).
7. MATHÉ, G., AMIEL, J. L., SCHWARZENBERG, L.: Bone marrow transplantation and leucocyte transfusions, 1 vol. Springfield, Ill.: C. C Thomas 1971.
8. MATHÉ, G., AMIEL, J. L., SCHWARZENBERG, L., HAYAT, M., DE VASSAL, F., SCHNEIDER, M., JASMIN, C., POUILLART, P.: Results of phase II clinical trials in the treatment of leukemias and lymphomas with epipodophyllotoxine derivatives, VM 26 and VP 16 213. In: 2. Arbeits. über Chemo- und Immunotherapie der Leukosen und malignen Lymphome. Vienne: March 1972.
9. MATHÉ, G., AMIEL, J. L., SCHWARZENBERG, L., SCHNEIDER, M., CATTAN, A., SCHLUMBERGER, J. R., HAYAT, M., DE VASSAL, F.: Active immunotherapy for acute lymphoid leukaemia. Lancet 1, 697. (1969).
10. MATHÉ, G., POUILLART, P., SCHWARZENBERG, L., AMIEL, J. L., SCHNEIDER, M., HAYAT, M., DE VASSAL, F., JASMIN, C., ROSENFIELD, C., WEINER, R., RAPPAPORT, H.: Attempts at immunotherapy of 100 acute lymphoid leukaemia patients. Some factors influencing results. Nat. Cancer Inst. Monogr. **35**, 361 (1972).
11. MATHÉ, G., RAPPAPORT, H.: Histological typing of the neoplastic diseases of the haematopoietic and lymphoid tissues. Genève: W.H.O. 1973, in press.
12. MILLER, J. F. A. P., MICHEL, G. F.: Cell to cell interaction in the immune responses. I. Hemolysin forming cells in neonatally thymectomized reconstituted with thymus or thoracic duct lymphocytes. J. exp. Med. **128**, 801 (1968).
13. MOORE, G. E., GRENER, R., FRANKLIN, A.: Culture of normal human leukocytes. J. Amer. med. Ass. **199**, 519 (1967).
14. PAINTRAND, M., DANTCHEV, D., MATHÉ, G.: Electron microscopic aspects of cells in the four sub-varieties of acute lymphoid leukemia. p. 71. In: Acute leukemias nomenclature, classification, clinical trials, methodology and actuarial results. G. MATHÉ, P. POUILLART and L. SCHWARZENBERG, eds., 1 vol. Berlin-Heidelberg-New York: Springer 1973.

15. PLUZNIK, D. H., SACHS, L.: The cloning of normal "mast" cells in tissue culture. J. cell. comp. Physiol. **66,** 319 (1965).
16. PLUZNIK, D. H., SACHS, L.: Induction of clones of normal "mast" cells by a substance from conditioned medium. Exp. Cell Res. **43,** 553 (1966).
17. POUILLART, P.: Contribution of cultures in agar to the classification of acute leukemias. p. 88. In: Acute leukemias nomenclature, classification, clinical trials, methodology and actuarial results. G. MATHÉ, P. POUILLART and L. SCHWARZENBERG, eds., 1 vol. Berlin-Heidelberg-New York: Springer 1973.
18. SIMONE, J. V., HOLLAND, E., JOHNSON, W.: Fatalities during remissions of childhood leukemia. Blood **39,** 759 (1972).

Classification of Acute Leukaemias Using Romanowsky, Sudan Black and Periodic Acid Schiff Stains

M. E. J. BEARD

Department of Haematology St. Bartholomew's Hospital, London/England

This report is based on four years' experience at St. Bartholomew's Hospital, London, during which 212 untreated cases of acute leukaemia were studied.

Table 1 states very briefly our criteria for subdividing these cases. In addition to ROMANOWSKY staining, we rely on two simple staining methods—Sudan black and the periodic acid Schiff reaction (P.A.S.). Sudan black allows positive identification of the myelogenous group. P.A.S. identifies the abnormal red-cell precursors usually found in erythroleukaemia as well as identifying most of the lymphoblastic group.

Using these criteria, we subdivided the cases as shown in Table 2. The application of these two cytochemical reactions to supplement ROMANOWSKY staining enabled us to classify 91% of cases by objective parameters. Only in the P.A.S.-negative group (6%) and the undifferentiated group (3%) did the precise diagnosis remain in doubt. Without these to additional reactions, the classification of 32.0% of our cases would have been uncertain and subjective; with them, the subjective element is reduced to 9%. Thus we believe that red (P.A.S.) or black (Sudan black) material in the cytoplasm, together with ROMANOWSKY staining, provides a much firmer basis for classification than ROMANOWSKY stains alone.

Table 1. Criteria for classifying the acute leukaemias

Myelogenous	
1. Myeloblastic	— Some or many blasts show coarse Sudan black positivity
2. Promyelocytic	— Predominant cell is the promyelocyte with heavy coarse granulation
3. Erythroleukaemia	— A myeloblastic component + > 40% abnormal red cell precursors, and/or strongly PAS-positive erythroblasts
4. Myelomonocytic	— "Significant" proportion of primitive cells monocytoid with fine Sudan black positivity
Lymphoblastic	
1. Definite	— Looks lymphoid; primitive cells PAS-positive (blocks)
2. Probable	— Looks lymphoid; primitive cells PAS-negative
Undifferentiated	
Primitive cells do not look lymphoid; PAS- and Sudan black-negative	

Table 2. Analysis of 212 cases of acute leukaemia

Myelogenous			
1. Myeloblastic	—	99 [10] [a]	(46.7%) [4.7] [a]
2. Promyelocytic	—	3	(1.4%)
3. Erythroleukaemia	—	4	(1.9%)
4. Myelomonocytic		38	(17.9%)
Lymphoblastic			
1. Definite	—	39	(18.4%)
2. Probable	—	13	(6.1%)
Undifferentiated	—	6	(2.8%)

[a] In these 10 cases their myeloblastic nature was uncertain on Romanowsky staining; correct diagnosis was made by Sudan black reaction.

Table 3 lists some of the problems that arise in classifying these cases. New techniques, perhaps to be discussed in this workshop, may lead to precise classification of all cases.

The lymphoid group remains difficult to subdivide mainly because few objective tests are available. The better prognosis of this group in children and the relation between disseminated and localized lymphoid tumours remains obscure. In the erythroleukaemias, if the P.A.S. reaction in the red-cell precursors is strongly positive, then B_{12}/folate therapy seems unnecessary. If the P.A.S is negative, or if there is any doubt over the diagnosis, then B_{12}/folate should be given for 1—2 weeks if practicable and the case then re-evaluated. The characterization of individual proliferating cell types should be made where possible, and the toluidine blue stain enables identification of any basophilic component that may be present.

In conclusion, the addition of two simple cytochemical methods greatly enhances the precision of Romanowsky staining. It makes the classification of acute leukaemias more objective and reproducible.

Table 3. Some problems in acute leukaemia classification

1. What is the nature of "probably lymphoid" and "undifferentiated" groups?
2. Is disseminated, poorly differentiated lymphocytic lymphoma identical morphologically to lymphoblastic leukaemia?
3. Should toluidine blue stain be used in myelogenous leukaemia to establish whether a basophilic component is present?
4. Should erythroleukaemia only be diagnosed after B_{12}/ folate therapy?
5. Does the degree of differentiation in the myeloblastic group correlate with survival?
6. In lymphoblastic leukaemia, why do children do better than adults?

Survival Prediction Based on Morphology of Lymphoblasts

J. M. BENNETT, M. R. KLEMPERER, and G. B. SEGEL

Departments of Medicine and Pediatries, The University of Rochester, School of Medicine and Dentistry, Division of Oncology and the Highland Hospital of Rochester, Rochester, NY/USA

Following publication of the paper entitled "Subdivision of Classical Varieties of Acute Leukemia. Correlation with Prognosis and Cure Expectancy" by G. MATHÉ *et al.* [1], considerable interest has been rekindled regarding the ability to 1. subclassify acute lymphocytic leukemia and 2. correlate the cell type with prognosis. The following study was an attempt to utilize the MATHÉ nomenclature of prolymphoblastic, macrolymphoblastic, microlymphoblastic, and prolymphocytic cell types in a series of acute lymphocytic leukemias of childhood (under 14 years of age) treated by the Pediatric-Hematology Unit of the University of Rochester School of Medicine.

Methods

Through the kind generosity of Professor MATHÉ, typical bone marrow smears of the subtypes were sent to one of us (J. M. B.). They were reviewed carefully and photographed (Figs. 1—4). Two hematologists (J. M. B. and G. B. S.) then defined

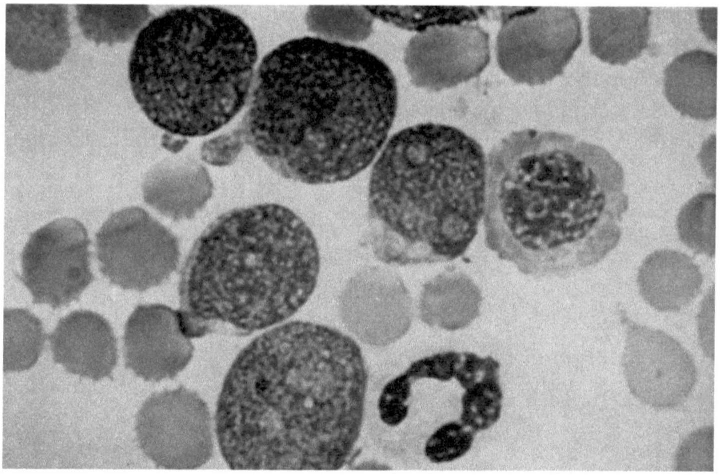

Fig. 1. Prolymphoblastic type

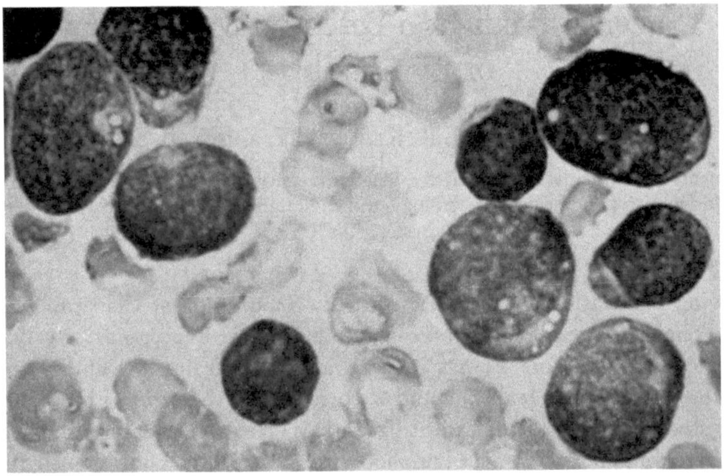

Fig. 2. Macrolymphoblastic type

criteria for the subtypes, following the classification of Mathé. The major features were: 1. size of cell, i.e. less than 12 micron in diameter for a microlymphoblast and greater than 12 micron for a macrolymphoblast; 2. chromatin pattern, i.e. very fine or reticulated for a prolymphoblast versus coarse pattern for a prolymphocyte; 3. grade of intensity of basophilic cytoplasm and amount, i.e. very basophilic with a lesser nucleo-cytoplasmic ratio for a prolymphoblast versus the blue-gray cytoplasm of a prolymphocyte; and 4. visibility of nucleoli, i.e. usually 1—2 in prolymphoblast versus 0—1 in other subtypes.

Cases of acute lymphocytic leukemia (A. L. L.) were then reviewed by a third hematologist (M. R. K.) who developed a series of 25 cases in which the original slides

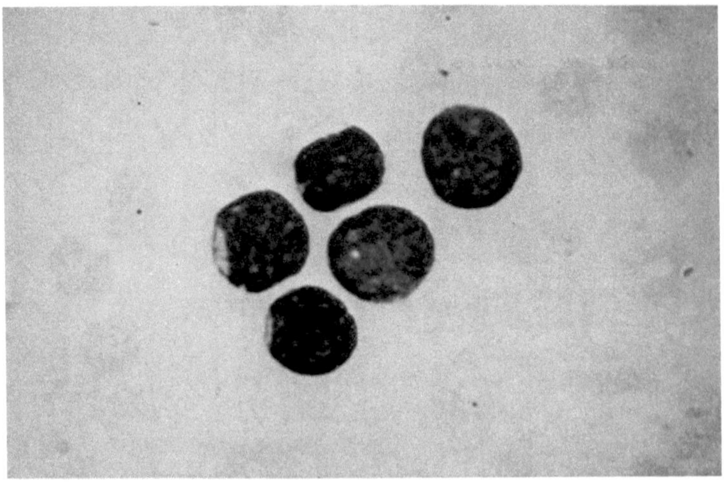

Fig. 3. Microlymphoblastic type

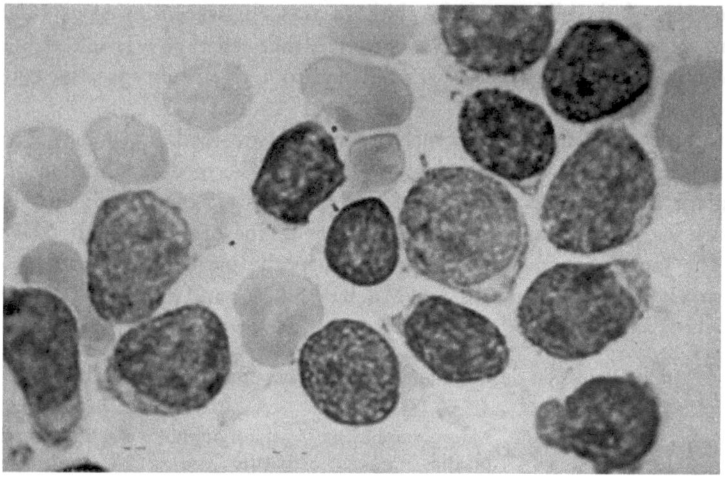

Fig. 4. Prolymphocytic type

were available and readily interpretable as A. L. L. morphologically and in some instances with P. A. S. and peroxidase stains. The slides were coded and read independently by J. M. B. and G. B. S. To test internal variability, the slides were recorded and reread two additional times.

Results

There was no significant difference between the two morphologists (J. M. B. and G. B. S.) in their internal consistency or ability to reproduce the same subtype classification when given the same slide three different times. One observer identified a given subtype three consecutive times (3 out of 3) in 12 cases, and 2 out of 3 times in 11 cases, whereas the other did likewise in 11 cases (3 out of 3) and 9 cases (2 out of 3), respectively. If one defines choosing a cell type 2 out of 3 or 3 out of 3 times as a reproducibility index (R. I.), then the R. I. for one observer was 92% and for the other 80%.

In 4 cases the cell type was called the same by both readers (microlymphoblastic in 3 and prolymphocytic in 1). In three cases, 5 out of 6 "calls" were the same (macrolymphoblastic in 2 and microlymphoblastic in 1). The R. I. was not improved by combining the observations of both readers (64%), indicating differences in individual interpretation of stained cells. This will be further commented on in this discussion. Neither observer identified a case as prolymphoblastic. The least degree of difficulty was experienced in identifying a case as either macro- or microlymphoblastic. Disagreements between macrolymphoblastic and prolymphocytic; prolymphocytic and microlymphoblastic; and inability to pick a single cell type more than once were evenly distributed.

Using the reproducibility index (R. I.) as a guide, all cases were reviewed together with a double-headed American Optical microscope. Areas on the glass slide were selected on a basis of — 1. thinness of preparation and normal erythrocytic morphology; 2. good contrast staining with the Wright's stain; and 3. avoiding the feathered edge, the sides of the slide, and the thick areas. Cells were viewed at 1000× magnification. If the agreement was 67% or better, that cell type was selected (16 cases). In the remaining 9 cases the slide was assigned to a given subtype after considerable discussion and debate.

Eight cases were classified as macrolymphoblastic (M.L.b.), 9 as microlymphoblastic (m.L.b.) and 8 as prolymphocytic (P.L.c.). The median duration of the first remission for M.L.b. was 7.5 months, for m.L.b. was 6.3 months, but for P.L.c. was 13.0, a strikingly significant difference in favor of the prolymphocytic cell type (see Table). The same phenomenon was apparent in the patient survival figures with a median survival of 16.0 months for M.L.b., 15.0 for m.L.b., and 23.0 months for P.L.c. Two of the long-term survivors are alive at 35+ and 52+ months and are both prolymphocytic. The oldest year of onset for the disease was 1961 and the most recent, 1970. No apparent difference in the mode of therapy for remission induction was noted, the majority of all patients receiving prednisone and 6-MP, or prednisone and methotrexate. Only two received prednisone and vincristine for induction.

Table. Remission duration and survival data in morphologic cell type

Cell type	Macrolympho-blastic	Microlympho-blastic	Prolympho-cytic
Number of cases	8	9	8
Available data	7	8	7
Duration of 1st remission (months)			
Mean	7.8	6.3	17.6
Median	7.5	6.3	13.0
Survival (months)			
Mean	18.4	15.5+	24.3+
Median	16.0	15.0	23.0

Discussion

For a new classification to be acceptable and of practical benefit, it must have a high degree of reproducibility and be fairly easily taught to other morphologist. Despite a lack of personal microscope instruction by Dr. Mathé, J. M. B. and G. B. S. achieved a high R. I. To complete the evaluation it would be necessary for the French group of Mathé *et al.* to classify our cases.

Disagreements either internal or between the two observers resulted in large measure from: 1. interpretation of cytoplasm as blue or blue-gray; 2. degree of nuclear clumping; and 3. cell size. Another key factor was the pleomorphism of cell type in several cases that resulted in an apparently significant percentage of 2 or more cell types. In 3 instances microlymphoblastic was the only cell type quickly identified 100% of the time.

Although the numbers are small, the prolonged survival of the prolymphocytic cell type is of interest. It was disappointing not to find a long survival in the microlymphoblastic group as well, but this may be a reflection of differences in treatment programs on the small numbers of cases evaluated to date.

In summary a double blind study of 25 cases of childhood acute lymphocytic leukemia were evaluated and classified according to the criteria of MATHÉ. Despite several problems a relatively high reproducibility index was obtained. No cases of prolymphoblastic leukemia were identified. A clear predominance of the prolymphocytic cell type was found in regard to both remission duration and survival.

References

1. MATHÉ, G., *et al.:* Subdivision of Classical Varieties of Acute Leukemia: Correlation with Prognosis and Cure Expectancy. Europ. J. clin. biol. Res. **16,** 554 (1971).

Cytology and Survival in Acute Lymphatic Leukemia of Children*

S. L. LEE and O. GLIDEWELL

Department of Medicine, Jewish Hospital Brooklin State University of New York Downstate, Medical Center Brooklyn, NY/USA

MATHÉ *et al.* (1971, 1972) have reported that children with acute lymphatic leukemia can be separated by a "technically simple classification" into four sub-types and that this classification correlates well with prognosis.

The Acute Leukemia Group B has been concerned for some time with the problem of the relationship between cytology and response to therapy in childhood leukemia. The data contained in the present report are offered in partial support of the evidence of MATHÉ *et al.* At the same time, the method of classification herein reported may possibly offer greater reliability and simplicity than that of MATHÉ.

Material and Methods

Patients included in this study were enrolled in Protocol 6313 of Acute Leukemia Group B (HOLLAND, 1968). All were under 21 years of age and were previously untreated. All patients seen with acute leukemia of any cell type were admitted to the study without selection. Microscopic slides of blood and bone marrow were sent to the Group Office, where their provenance was recorded and they were given an identification number. The slides were stained with Wright-Giemsa or May-Gruenwald-Giemsa and delivered to a single observer (SLL), to whom they were identified only by number. Of 187 patients entered in the study, satisfactory slides were obtained and examined in 170 cases. Seventeen patients were diagnosed by both the original observer and by the reviewer as having acute myeloblastic leukemia. The remaining 153 cases of acute lymphatic leukemia form the subject material of the present report.

Slides were examined and rated numerically for criteria which in a previous study (LEE *et al.*, 1962) had been found useful for identifying acute lymphatic leukemia. These criteria were (A) presence of azurophilic granules (punctate or coarse); (B) amount of cytoplasm relative to size of nucleus; (C) prominence of nucleoli in leukemic cells. In most instances bone marrow smears were used for these determinations, although in occasional cases the peripheral blood smear furnished the best preserved examples of leukemic cells.

* Supported by grants (CA-05923, CA-12286, CA-10456) from the National Cancer Institutes of Health.

Quantitation of Morphologic Criteria

A. Azurophil granules. Were scored as *0* (absent), *1* (few granules in a minority of cells judged to be leukemic) or *2* (many granules in a minority of leukemic cells or any granules in more than 50% of leukemic cells). No attempt was made to differentiate fine dust-like granulation from coarse, larger granules in this classification.

B. Amount of cytoplasm visible. Was scored as *0* (virtually none), *1* (thin rim) or *2* (larger quantities). The value assigned for this criterion represented an average of at least 50 leukemic cells.

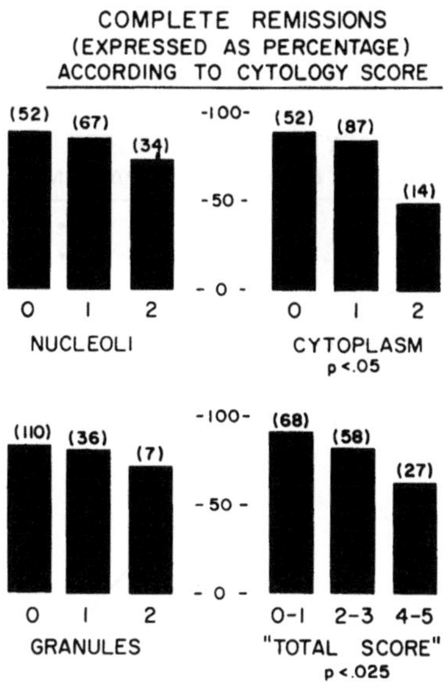

Fig. 1. Complete remissions (expressed as percentage) according to cytology score for *nucleoli*, *cytoplasm*, *granules* and all of these combined ("total score"). The number in parentheses above each bar represents the number of patients in each grouping. Where "p" values are not indicated, they are greater than 0.05

C. Number and prominence of nucleoli in leukemic cells. Was scored as *0* (none visible), *1* (one of moderate size per cell) or *2* (especially large or prominent or more than one per cell). The number recorded represented the mean (to the nearest whole number) of at least 50 cells.

Other cytologic characteristics. Degree of fineness (dispersion) of the chromatin network, presence of vacuoles, proportion of norma-appearing granulocytic and erythropoietic elements—were also examined and scored. However, since grading of these characteristics did not appear to improve significantly the prognostic significance of the cytologic studies, they will not be discussed further.

Cytology scores for each of the three criteria were correlated with attainment of complete remission after the protocol therapy and with survival from the time of diagnosis. Standard statistical methods were used.

Results

Complete Remission (Fig. 1).

Fig. 1 demonstrates that for all three cytologic characteristics the proportion of complete remissions decreased as the individual score mounted. This relationship was statistically significant only in the case of *cytoplasm.*

Summation of the scores for each characteristic for each patient puts the correlation between "total score" and percentage of complete remissions on a much firmer statistical basis. Of the 27 patients with a "total score" of four or five, only 63% achieved remission, while 90% of the 68 whose "total score" was zero or one reached that status.

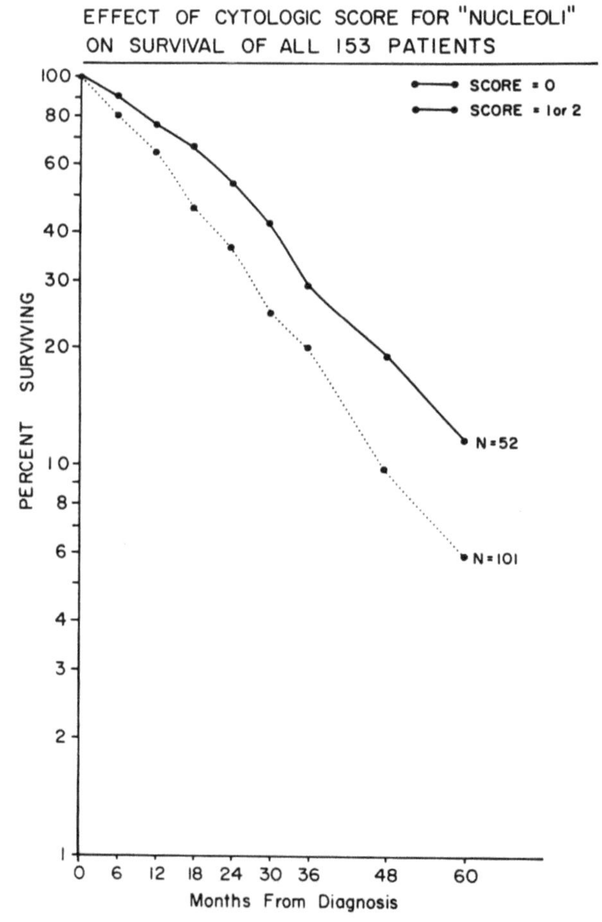

Fig. 2. Effect of cytology score for *nucleoli* on the survival of all 153 patients with acute lymphoid leukemia. The solid line represents the actuarial survival curve for the 52 patients whose score was zero. The dotted line represents the actuarial curve for the remaining 101 patients

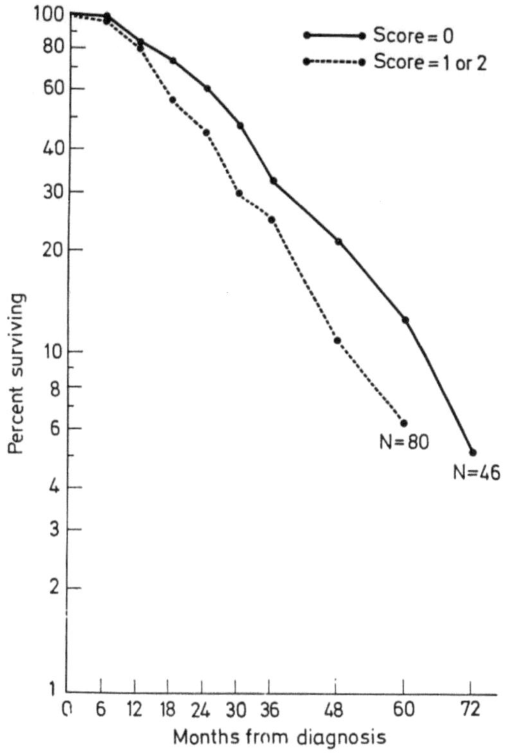

Fig. 3. Effect of cytology score for *nucleoli* on the survival of the 126 patients who achieved complete remission

Survival

Survival from the time of diagnosis was calculated for each score group for each cytologic characteristic. In spite of the observed differences in remission rates, no significant survival differences were observed except in the case of the *nucleoli.* Fifty-two patients with *nucleoli* score of zero had a median survival of 26 months; 101 with higher scores had a median survival of 17 months. The curves shown in Fig. 2 differ significantly at the 0.05 level of confidence by the Breslow test. Fig. 3 shows that the difference persists even when comparison is limited to patients who achieved complete remission.

For cytoplasm, (Fig. 4) and for granules (Fig. 5) the actuarial curves do not vary significantly with morphology score, nor do the median survival times of the patient groups. Survival could not be shown to relate to either of these cytologic criteria, whether all 153 patients or the 126 achieving complete remission were considered.

Discussion

These studies appear to show that, in acute lymphoblastic leukemia of children, the cytologic characteristics, cytoplasm, granules and nucleoli correlate with the probability of complete remission after treatment with prednisone and vincristine. These

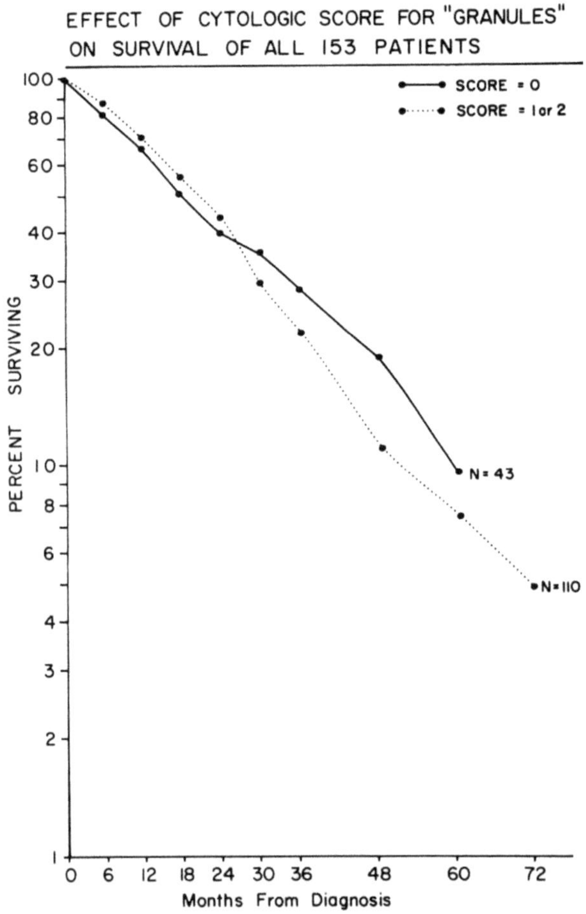

Fig. 4. Effect of cytology score for granules on the survival of all 153 patients. The solid line represents the actuarial survival curve for the 43 patients whose score was zero. The dotted line represents the actuarial curve for the remaining 110 patients. These curves are not significantly

characteristics are the very same ones which, in a previous study (Lee *et al.*, 1962) as well as in another part of the analysis of the present study (Lee and Glidewell, unpublished) served best to differentiate the myeloblast of acute myeloblastic leukemia from the lymphoblast of acute lymphoblastic leukemia. Thus those patients with acute lymphoblastic leukemia whose leukemic cells most resembled myeloblasts (while still remaining recognizably lymphoblasts) had a lower rate of remission than did those patients whose leukemic cells were least like myeloblasts (Fig. 1).

Mathé *et al.* (1971) have looked at the degree of reticulation of *chromatin*, prominence of *nucleoli*, amount of *cytoplasm*, and *size of leukemic cells* in a group of 45 patients under 20 years of age with acute lymphoblastic leukemia (all patients having achieved complete remission). They separated four cytologic sub-types:—prolymphoblastic, macrolymphoblastic, prolymphocytic and microlymphoblastic with

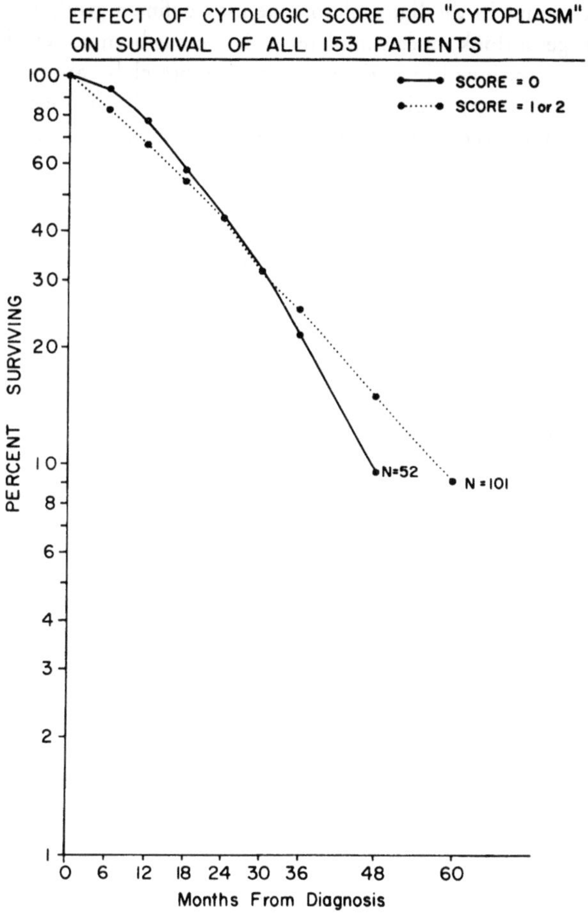

Fig. 5. Effect of cytology score for *cytoplasm* on the survival of all 153 patients. The solid line represents the actuarial survival curve for the 52 patients whose score was zero. The dotted line represents the actuarial curve for the remaining 101 patients. These curves were not significantly different

progressively better survival in that order. Nucleolar prominence apparently distinguished the group with the worst prognosis—the prolymphoblastic.

The present series, in a larger number of patients, also appears to demonstrate that prominent nucleoli in leukemic lymphoblasts signal shorter survival (Figs. 2 and 3), and thus partly confirms the findings of MATHÉ *et al.* The scoring system here reported has served to analyzc the effects on survival of five different cytologic characteristics, including all those used by MATHÉ *et al.* except for cell size. None except *nucleoli* could be shown to correlate at all with patient survival.

These data suggest that the present classification of children with acute lymphoblastic leukemia into four subcategories for prognostic purposes is not warranted. Identification of patients whose cells have very inconspicuous nucleoli when viewed with ROMANOWSKY stains in the light microscope may define a group of patients with a better-than-average outlook, once complete remission has been achieved.

Studies are being continued in patients receiving more elaborate (and presumably more effective) chemotherapy regimens. It is hoped that sub-categorization by cytologic characteristics will eventually permit more intelligent therapeutic management.

References

HOLLAND, J. F.: Progress in the Treatment of Acute Leukemia, 1966. p. 217. In: DAMESHEK, W., DUTCHER, R. M., eds.: Perspectives in leukemia. New York: Grune & Stratton 1968.

LEE, S. L., GLIDEWELL, O.: Unpublished data.

LEE, S. L., LIVINGS, D., JAMES, G. W., SCHROEDER, L., SELAWRY, O., STICKNEY, J. M.: Morphologic classification of acute leukemias. Cancer Chemother. Rep. **16**, 151 (1962).

MATHÉ, G., AMIEL, J. L., SCHWARZENBERG, L., SCHNEIDER, M., HAYAT, M., DE VASSAL, F., POUILLART, P.: Attempts at stimulation of immune response in acute lymphoid leukemia. Proc. roy. Soc. Med. **65**, 266 (1972).

MATHÉ, G., POUILLART, P., STERESCU, M., AMIEL, J. L., SCHWARZENBERG, L., SCHNEIDER, M., HAYAT, M., DE VASSAL, F., JASMIN, C., LAFLEUR, M.: Subdivision of classical varieties of acute leukemia. Correlation with prognosis and cure expectancy. Europ. J. clin. biol. Res. **16**, 554 (1971).

Histologic Criteria for Diagnosis and Classification of Acute Leukemias*

H. RAPPAPORT

Institut de Cancérologie et d'Immunogénétique, Villejuif/France and
The University of Chicago, Chicago, IL/USA

As a rule, acute leukemias are diagnosed and classified on the basis of Wright or Giemsa-stained blood and bone marrow smears. When a good marrow sample is obtained, histologic study of the tissue sections only rarely contributes to the diagnosis or classification. There are certain circumstances, however, under which histologic study of tissue sections may be essential to the diagnosis of acute leukemia. This is usually the case in the aleukemic patient when the marrow smear is poor in cells and some of these cells appear immature without being readily classifiable, or when a biopsy from an extramedullary lesion precedes a bone marrow study or is taken at a time when clear-cut leukemic changes in the bone marrow are not evident.

In the first instance, there is usually uncertainty as to whether the lack of nucleated cellular elements of the bone marrow smear is due to technical problems leading to hemodilution, or whether the hypocellular sample represents the true state of the bone marrow. This can always be resolved by a representative bone marrow section which may either disclose a marrow full of blast cells (Fig. 1) without apparent reason for the hemodilution in routinely stained sections, or a truly hypocellular marrow indicative of a hyporegenerative anemia. The reason why a cellular marrow may consistently yield a hypocellular sample is not always clear. In my experience one can, in most such instances, demonstrate by proper staining methods an increase in reticulin fibers (Fig. 2). These impart to the bone marrow a cohesiveness which the negative pressure in the aspirating needle cannot overcome. When the bone marrow is cellular and completely infiltrated with immature forms (Fig. 3), histologic sections usually do not disclose the type of leukemia, and it is always important to obtain, at the time when the surgical biopsy is performed, imprints which can be stained by the Wright (Fig. 4) or Giemsa methods. Once imprints are available, the problems of classifications which occur are the same as those in cellular marrow smears obtained by aspiration [3]. In acute myeloid leukemia occasional eosinophilic myelocytes may be recognized in tissue sections. This is, however, more common in extramedullary localization and will be discussed below.

---

* Supported, in part, by Grant No. CA-05838, from the National Cancer Institute, National Institutes of Health.

When the presence of a hypocellular marrow is confirmed histologically, this will almost always be a strong indication that one is dealing with hyporegenerative anemia rather than an acute leukemia. Occasionally, however, one may not be able to decide between a hyporegenerative anemia and a so-called preleukemic phase of acute leukemia. A predominance of blast cells points in the direction of leukemia. Karyotype analysis has not always been helpful in doubtful cases [5]. As a rule, only the evolution of the disease allows one to make this decision eventually.

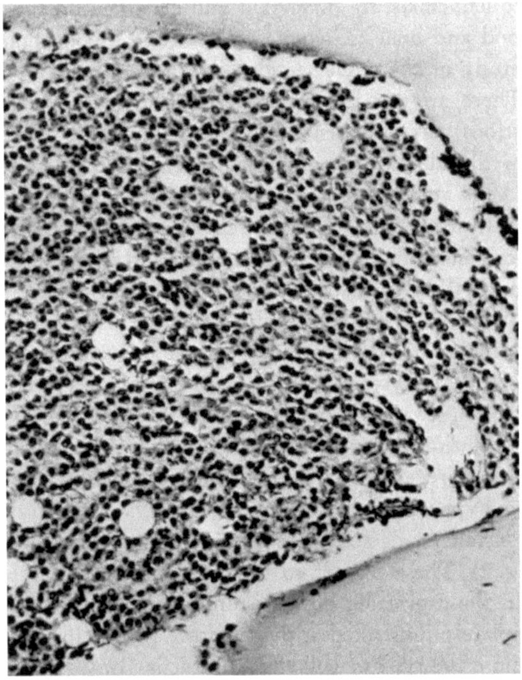

Fig. 1. Bone marrow — Acute myeloid leukemia. In this histologic section from the biopsy specimen, note the uniform, diffuse cellular proliferation and the scarcity of marrow fat. Hematoxylin and eosin stain. ×200

In extramedullary localization, histologic study is often the only method available for diagnosis and at times for the classification of an acute leukemia. A biopsy may be performed under the following circumstances: 1. A patient without known leukemia may have lymph node enlargement, or a skin lesion, or an extramedullary tumor, and histologic study is the first examination which results in the diagnosis of acute leukemia. 2. In patients with known acute leukemia, a biopsy of an extramedullary lesion is performed for the purpose of establishing whether or not it is part of the leukemic disease, or a complication of it, or an unrelated lesion.

In acute lymphoid leukemias, lymph node enlargement may be the first manifestation of the disease, but is usually preceded by other symptoms and signs attributable to a pancytopenic state. However, on occasion the pathologist is presented with an excised lymph node and may find it difficult to distinguish between malignant lymphoma of the poorly differentiated lymphocytic type (lymphosarcoma) and acute lymphoid (lymphoblastic) leukemia. This distinction is at times possible from technically perfect tissue sections alone. Usually, however, the histologic diagnosis of acute lymphoid leukemia is tentative and subject to confirmation by appropriate Wright or Giemsa stains, either of lymph node imprints or of smears of bone marrow or blood. In tissue sections, the blast cells of acute lymphoid leukemia (Fig. 5) are more

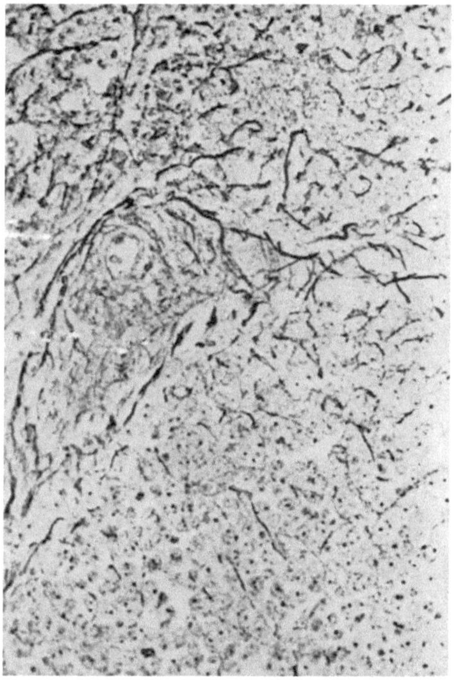

Fig. 2. Bone marrow — Acute myeloid leukemia (same case as Fig. 1). The obvious increase of reticulin fibers in this bone marrow probably accounts for the difficulty in obtaining a cellular marrow sample by aspiration; the fibers may cause a cohesiveness of the marrow tissue that cannot be overcome by the negative pressure in the aspirating needle. Silver impregnation for reticulin; method of SNOOK. ×300

uniform and have more delicate chromatin structure and small and relatively indistinct nucleoli [4]. The cells of poorly differentiated lymphosarcoma show considerable variations in nuclear size, shape and staining quality, and a much coarser chromatin structure with rather distinct nucleoli. In acute lymphoid leukemias, atypical reticulum cells are rare, whereas in poorly differentiated lymphosarcomas they are scattered through the sections in appreciable numbers. When the acute lymphoid leukemia is of the prolymphocytic type [3], histologic or even cytologic differentiation from malignant lymphoma of the poorly differentiated lymphocytic-type sarcoma may be impossible. The best single differential diagnostic feature, in my experience, is the presence of thrombocytopenia in acute lymphoid leukemias even during the early clinical phases of the disease, while in "leukemic lymphosarcoma," thrombocytopenia may be either moderate or lacking even when lymph node enlargement is pronounced.

Other acute leukemias are rarely diagnosed from lymph node sections alone. In the occasional case where a lymph node biopsy is available in an acute myeloid or monocytoid leukemia, the complete obliteration of the architecture that one sees in

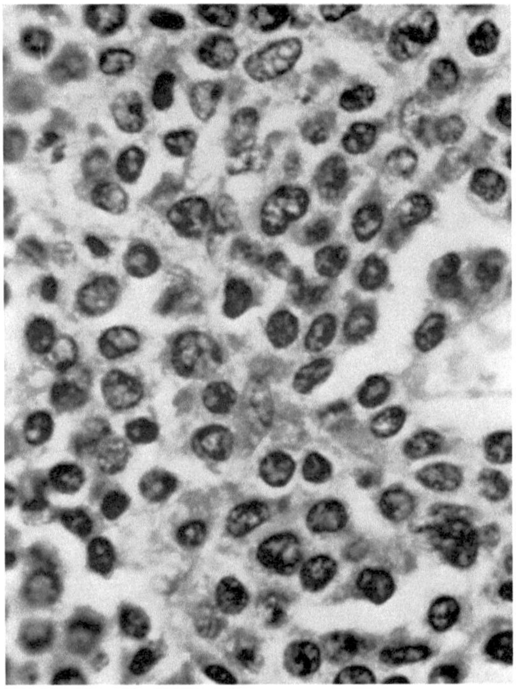

Fig. 3. Bone marrow — Acute myeloid leukemia (same case as Fig. 1). At higher magnification, note the relative uniformity of the proliferating cells; their nuclei vary only moderately in size and shape. Since positive identification of these undifferentiated cells as myeloblasts is usually not possible from histologic sections, imprints from the biopsy specimen should be done; such preparations may be of value in establishing an unequivocal diagnosis (Fig. 4). Hematoxylin and eosin stain. ×1000

most instances of acute lymphoid leukemia is not evident. A few islands of normal-appearing lymphocytes are often preserved. In acute monocytoid leukemias the monocytes are often recognizable by their deeply indented nuclei which are particularly well demonstrable with fine focusing at various levels of the nucleus [1]. In the acute myeloid leukemias, one often sees eosinophilic myelocytes (Fig. 7) which actually offer a key for the diagnosis in tissue sections, since neutrophilic granules are not seen in hematoxylin- and eosin-stained sections, and basophilic granules are readily dissolved in aqueous fixatives. One therefore depends on the eosinophilic myelocytes for recognition of other cells with similar nuclei as immature elements of the myeloid series. Lymph node enlargement due to myeloid proliferation may occur in chronic myeloid leukemia at the time of blast crisis. Sections from such large lymph nodes are at times mistaken for "reticulum-cell sarcoma" or other malignant lymphomas, and the existence of two diseases is postulated. This diagnostic pitfall can be avoided either by the appreciation of the importance of the eosiniphilic myelocytes or by the demonstration of a non-specific esterase by the naphthol-AS-D-chloracetate esterase method [2].

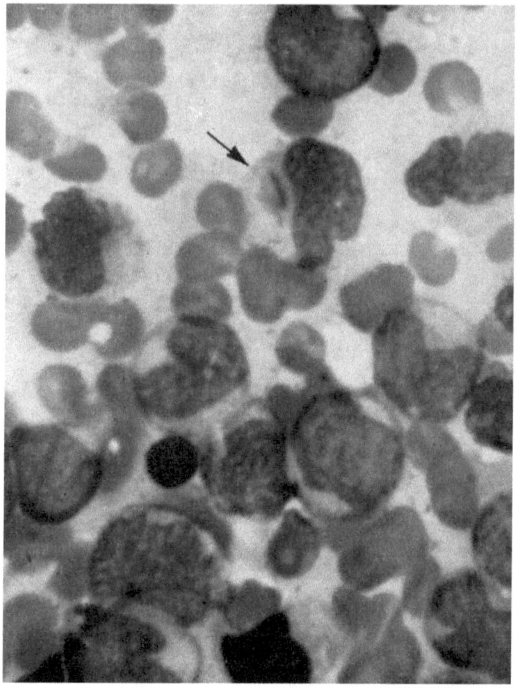

Fig. 4. Bone marrow — Acute myeloid leukemia (same case as Fig. 1). This bone marrow imprint was made from the biopsy specimen immediately after surgery. It shows slightly distorted immature cells; since one of these (arrow) contains an Auer body, acute myeloid leukemia was readily diagnosed. Wright-Giemsa stain. ×1100

Other extramedullary localizations of the acute leukemias are the skin, particularly in the acute monocytoid leukemias, the subperiosteal tissues, particularly in the myeloid (granulocytic) sarcomas (so-called chloromas), and the gonads. Less common locations are the breast and the subcutaneous tissue. The myeloid sarcomas may at times become evident before the diagnosis of acute myeloid leukemia can be made with certainty from the bone marrow and peripheral blood. I have, however, only followed one case in which evidence of acute leukemia did not appear within one year following the appearance of the extramedullary tumors; this patient was a child with a myeloid sarcoma of the maxillary antrum who is still alive and without diagnosable leukemia three years after appearance of the tumor.

The histologic diagnosis of acute leukemia in sections of gonads is particularly significant since gonadal involvement may be observed in treated and otherwise asymptomatic patients with acute lymphoid leukemia who have been well controlled therapeutically for many years. These gonadal recurrences are almost always observed in the lymphoid leukemias, more specifically in those of the prolymphocytic type, and are histologically indistinguishable from poorly differentiated lymphosarcomas. This is not surprising since both cytologically and histologically a clear-cut dif-

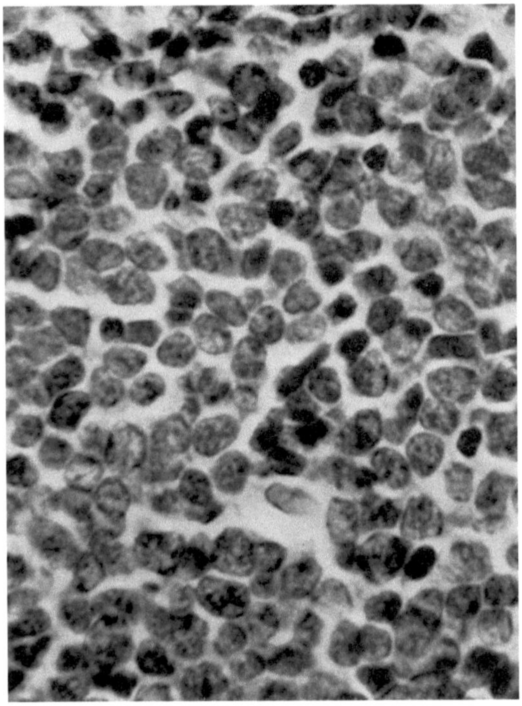

Fig. 5. Lymph node — Acute lymphoid leukemia. In comparison with Fig. 6, the variations in the nuclear size and shape are slight; the nuclei have fine, delicate chromatin structures. The nucleoli are small and are often indistinct. Although the identification of these immature cells as lymphoid cells is impossible from tissue sections, they can be distinguished from the lymphocytes of poorly differentiated lymphosarcoma (malignant lymphoma, poorly differentiated lymphocytic type). Hematoxylin and eosin stain. ×100

ferentiation between poorly differentiated lymphosarcoma and prolymphocytic lymphoid leukemia may be exceedingly difficult, if not impossible, morphologically.

In summary, I wish to say that, in the great majority of cases, histologic studies are not necessary either to establish the presence of a leukemic process or to classify it. However, in rare instances, a definitive diagnosis has to depend on a histologic study, particularly in the pancytopenic patient from whom it is impossible to obtain an adequate marrow sample by aspiration. Occasionally a biopsy from an extramedullary lesion may provide the first indication of the presence of acute leukemia.

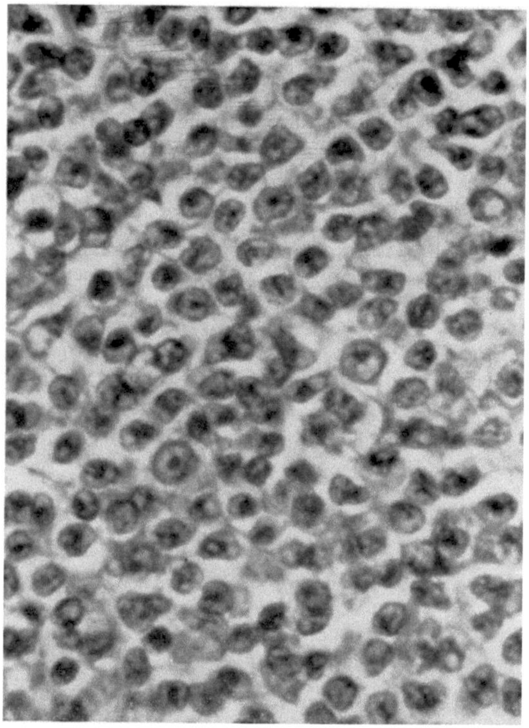

Fig. 6. Lymph node — Malignant lymphoma, poorly differentiated lymphocytic type (poorly differentiated lymphosarcoma). The majority of the proliferating atypical cells are neoplastic lymphocytes; their nuclei show marked variations in size and shape. Also note the presence of larger cells, so-called malignant reticulum cells (center). These cells have larger nuclei, thicker nuclear membranes, and larger, more prominent nucleoli than the proliferating lymphocytes. They are often present in small to moderate numbers in this type of malignant lymphoma. Hematoxylin and eosin stain. ×1000

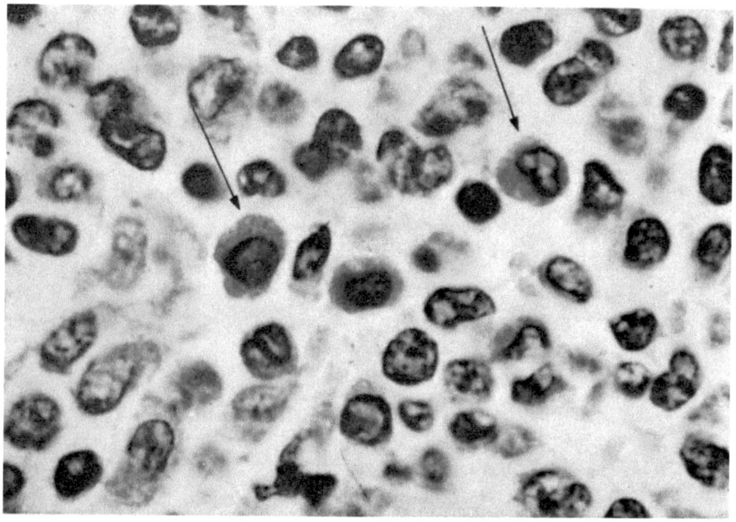

Fig. 7. Testis — Myeloid (granulocytic) sarcoma. An abnormal proliferation of hematopoietic cells that could be easily confused with reticulum cell sarcoma or lymphosarcoma were it not for the presence of two eosinophilic myelocytes (arrows). Hematoxylin and eosin stain. ×1000

References

1. FORKNER, C. E.: Clinical and pathologic differentiation of the acute leukemias. With special reference to acute monocytic leukemia. Arch. intern. Med. **53**, 1 (1934).
2. LEDER, L. D.: Der Nachweis der Naphthol-AS-D-Chloracetat-Esterase und seine Bedeutung für die histologische Diagnostik. Verh. dtsch. path. Ges. **48**, 317 (1964).
3. MATHÉ, G., POUILLART, P., STERESCU, M., AMIEL, J. L., SCHWARZENBERG, L., SCHNEIDER, M., HAYAT, M., DE VASSAL, F., JASMIN, C., LAFLEUR, M.: Subdivision of classical varieties of acute leukemia. Correlation with prognosis and cure expectancy. Europ. J. clin. biol. Res. **16**, 554 (1971).
4. RAPPAPORT, H.: Tumors of the hematopoietic system, p. 22. Washington, D. C., 1966, Armed Forces Institute of Pathology.
5. ROWLEY, J., BLAISDELL, R. K., JACOBSON, L. O.: Chromosome studies in preleukemia. Blood **27**, 782 (1966)

Practical Value of Cytochemical Studies for the Classification of Acute Leukemias

G. Flandrin and M. T. Daniel

Institut de Recherches sur les Leucémies et les Maladies du Sang, Hôpital Saint-Louis, Paris/France

The cell variety in acute leukemia (AL) may be difficult to identify when the examination of blood and marrow is restricted to May-Grunwald-Giemsa (MGG) staining methods. (II) Various cytochemical techniques have been used [1, 4, 5, 11, 12, 13, 14, 15, 18, 19, 20]. These methods have been shown to provide a valuable approach to demonstrating characteristic features of abnormal cell lines.

However, opinions differ as to the utility of the different reactions. We have studied several hundred patients with acute leukemia by both cytological and cytochemical methods in order to gather information on the practical value of the various cytochemical reactions.

Material and Methods

From January 1968 to May 1972, 921 patients with AL were studied in our laboratory (Table 1). These cases were first classified by MGG according to classical cytological criteria [17]. During 1968 and 1969, peroxidase and periodic acid Schiff (PAS) reactions were systematically performed. Thereafter, cytochemical reactions were done only when cytological difficulties were encountered. The cytochemical

Table 1. Total of AL patients studied 1968—1972 Hôpital Saint-Louis — Paris

	1968	1969	1970	1971	1972 [a]	Total
Acute lymphoblastic leukemia	93	91	87	53	42	366
Acute non-lymphoblastic leukemia	139	107	121	148	40	555 [b]
Total	232	198	208	201	82	921

[a] Study ended May 1972 —
[b] Includes AGL — 33 acute promyelocytic
— 14 acute monocytic (since 1970)
— 24 unclassifiable (or undifferentiated) acute leukemias.

reactions used are the following: PAS [10], naphthol AS-D chloroacetate esterase [19, 20] and naphthol AS-D acetate esterase [5, 14].

The value of naphthol AS-D acetate esterase inhibition by 1.5 mg/ml sodium fluoride in diagnosing acute monocytic leukemia had been previously demonstrated in 40 acute leukemia cases. We have been using this technique routinely since 1970 whenever acute monocytic leukemia is suspected.

Patients with blastic crises of chronic myeloproliferative disorders (chronic myeloid leukemia, myelofibrosis with myeloid metaplasia polycythemia) were excluded from this study, as well as the occasional leukemic picture which may occur in malignant histiocytosis.

Results: PAS Reaction

PAS Reaction in Acute Lymphoblastic Leukemia (ALL)

The PAS reaction was studied in 100 cases (Table 2). In 43 patients blast cells were first thought to be PAS-negative. However, after careful scanning of the slides, in 19 cases a very few positive blast cells were observed, less than 1% in all instances, with a discrete, fine granular pattern of positivity. In the 24 remaining patients, no positive cells were found in spite of repeated careful examination.

Eleven other patients had a fine, regularly scattered, granular pattern of positivity which was easy to identify on the slide (Fig. 1 a).

The 46 remaining cases had coarse granules of PAS-positive material, often a single one close to the edge of the cell or projecting over the nucleus when there was a narrow cytoplasmic rim. This pattern was very typical of ALL; in other examples the PAS positivity was heavy with numerous fine and coarse granules and sometimes heavy blocks of positivity (Fig. 1 b).

All the cases with a very high percentage of PAS-positive blast cells belonged to this group with "typical" coarse granules of positive material (see Table 3).

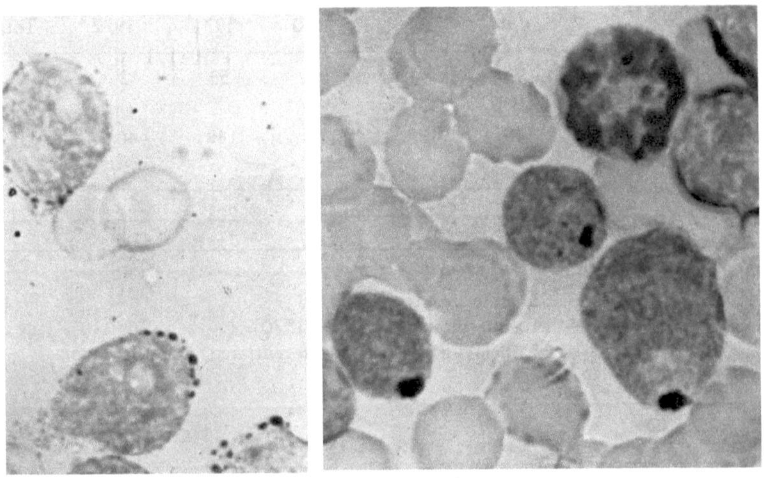

a b

Fig. 1 a and b. Acute lymphoblastic leukemia — PAS reaction. a Fine granular pattern positivity, b Coarse "typical" granular positivity

Table 2. Ratio of children to adults among the AL patients shown in Table 1

	Acute lymphoblastic leukemia		Acute non-lymphoblastic leukemia	
	Children under 18	Adults	Children under 18	Adults
1968	83	10	25	114
1969	80	11	26	81
1970	66	21	14	107
1971	46	7	25	123
1972 [a]	30	12	12	28
	305	61	102	453

[a] Study ended May 1972.

Table 3. PAS reaction in ALL patients

	PAS negativity (or less than 1% positive)	PAS positivity	
		Fine granular pattern [c]	"Typical" coarse granular pattern [b]
No. of cases	43 [c]	11	46
% of PAS-positive blast cells	—	Average 6% Range 2 to 39%	Average 38% Range 2 to 100%

[a] Fine granular positivity only.

[b] Variable positivity ranging from fine to coarse granules and blocks; coarse granules predominant.

[c] 24 cases showed complete negativity, and 19 cases had less than 1% of cells with a discrete fine granular pattern.

Table 4. Cytological correlation in attempt ED classification of ALL from Mathé [16] [a]

Cytological subclasses	Three observers agreed no. of cases	Two observers agreed (third observer's classification in parenthesis) no. of cases	Total cases
Subclass 1 prolymphoblastic	18	6 (6 with subclass 2)	24
Subclass 2 macrolymphoblastic	32	15 (8 with subclass 1) (7 with subclass 3)	47
Subclass 3 microlymphoblastic	12	6 (6 with subclass 2)	18
Subclass 4 prolymphocytic	5	3 (1 with subclass 1) (1 with subclass 2) (1 with subclass 3)	8

[a] Note: There were 4 cases where all three observers disagreed; there were omitted from the study.

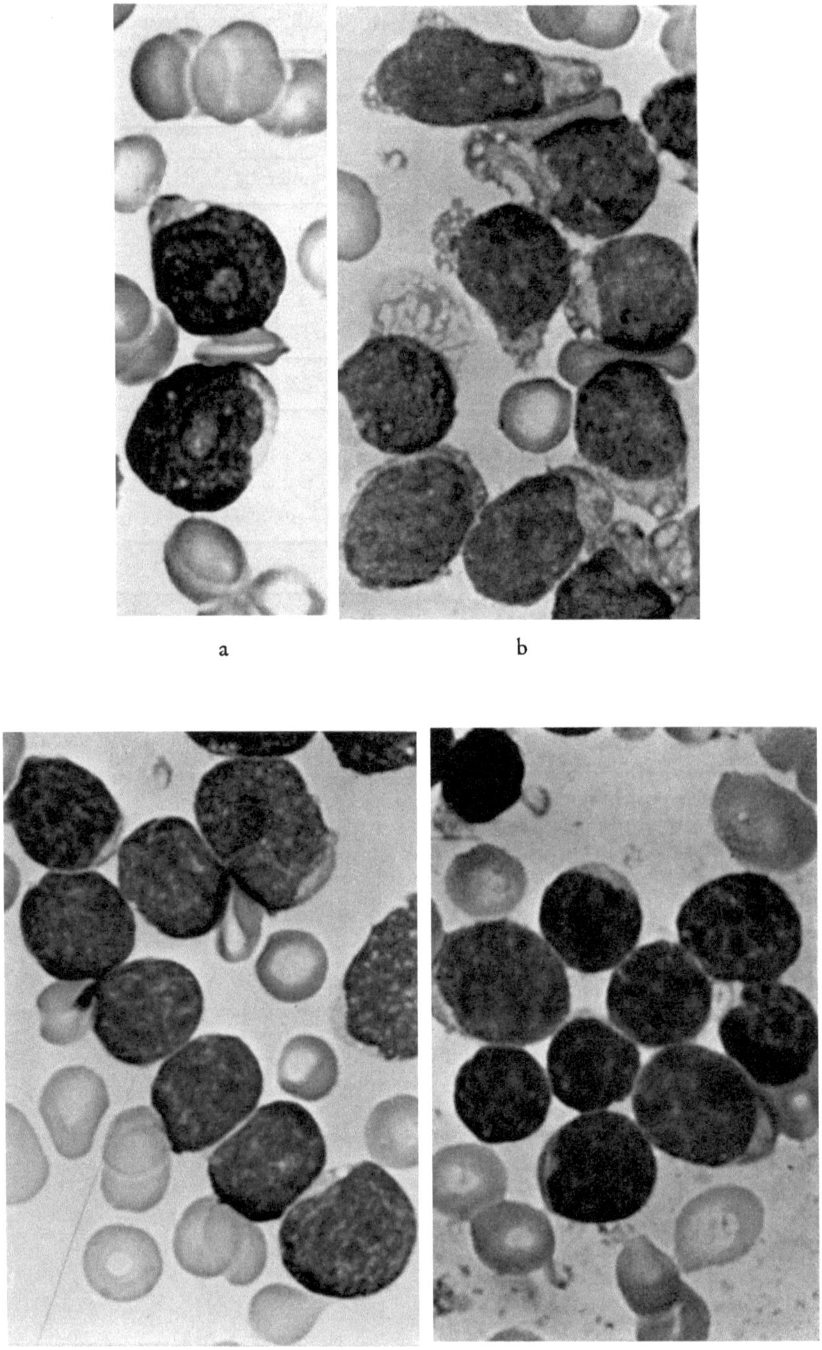

a b

c d

Fig. 2 a—d. Acute lymphoblastic leukemia — Cytological subclasses from MATHÉ's classification. a Subclass 1 (prolymphoblastic), b Subclass 2 (macrolymphoblastic), c Subclass 3 (microlymphoblastic), d Subclass 4 (prolymphocytic)

In keeping with recent attempts by Mathé *et al.* [16] to propose a new sub-classification of ALL into four groups, we have found several differences between patients in 100 cases (Fig. 2 a—d and Table 4).

We tried to correlate this cytological sub-classification with our results obtained with PAS reaction in the same cases. Our ability to reproduce the Mathé's sub-classification was not absolute. In double-blind trials we found, after three observers had examined these 100 cases, that all three failed to agree in about one third of the cases. Nevertheless, there were four cases remained where all three disagreed and they were excluded from the study. Some confusion did exist between subclass 2, on the one hand and subclasses 1 or 3 on the other hand. We accepted only agreement in double-blind tests as sufficient evidence for classification.

The correlation of this ALL sub-classification with our PAS-reaction results is not strikingly obvious (Table 5). However, the ratio of "typical" coarse-granule pattern

Table 5. Correlation of cytological subclasses of ALL with results of PAS reaction in blast cells

	Subclass 1 no. of cases	Subclass 2 no. of cases	Subclass 3 no. of cases	Subclass 4 no. of cases
PAS-negative or less than 1%	11	22	7	2
PAS-positive fine granular pattern	7	1	1	0
PAS-positive "typical" coarse-granule pattern	6	23	10	6

Table 6. PAS positivity in blast cells and average age of patient

	No. of cases	Children under 18		No. of cases	Adults over 18		No. of cases	All cases [c]	
		Average age yrs	Range		Average age yrs	Range		Average age yrs	Range
PAS negativity or less than 1%	35	7	1 to 17	8	35	20 to 64	43	12	1 to 67
PAS positivity fine granular pattern	6	7	2 to 15	5	63	45 to 74	11	33	2 to 74
PAS positivity [b] Coarse granules "typical" pattern	36	6	1 to 17	10	43	21 to 61	46	15	1 to 61

[a] Complete PAS negativity (24 cases) and less than 1% positive blast cells (19) of the fine granular pattern type.

[b] 14 of these cases had more than 60% PAS-positive blast cells in their bone marrow.

[c] Average age of the whole group of 100 ALL patients = 15 years (median 8 years).

to the other PAS-positive pattern was lower in subclass 1 than in the others, (1 : 3 in subclass 1, and about 1 : 1 in subclasses 2 and 3; 4 is a too small sample for any correlation).

It may be noted that there were as many children as adults in the fine-granular-pattern PAS-positive group, whereas there were four times more children than adults in the other two groups (Table 6). The overall ratio of adults to children with ALL may be recalled here (Table 2).

If one now compares the age distribution of the different cytological subgroups, according to Mathé's criteria, there are found to be nearly twice as many children as adults in subclass 1; this picture was quite different in the other subclasses (Table 7).

Table 7. ALL subclasses and average age of the patients

	No. of cases	Children under 18		No. of cases	Adults over 18		No. of cases	ALL cases	
		Average age yrs	Range		Average age yrs	Range		Average age yrs	Range
ALL subclass 1	15	8	2 to 16	9	47	21 to 74	24	22	2 to 74
ALL subclass 2	40	7	1 to 17	7	40	20 to 55	47	12	1 to 55
ALL subclass 3	14	5	1 to 15	4	42	26 to 61	18	15	1 to 61
ALL subclass 4	6	3	1 to 6	one case only	64				

PAS Reaction and Acute Nonlymphoblastic Leukemias

Acute Granulocytic Leukemia

The typical single coarse-granule pattern of some forms of ALL was never seen in AGL.

More frequently, PAS reaction was negative in all the blast cells of AGL. PAS positivity was seen in about one third of the cases of AGL in a varying number of cells. In these cases, it was sometimes very difficult to differentiate between myeloblasts and maturing granulocytic cells which were normally PAS-positive. When the PAS reaction was positive in myeloblasts, this positivity ranged from a weak diffused rim over most of the cytoplasm to occasional areas of increases smooth, fine granularity.

Acute Monocytic Leukemia

Monocytic precursors showed great variability in their PAS reaction, ranging from negative cells to fine or moderate granular positivity, regularly scattered in the cytoplasm. Of 11 cases studied, we found only one where the blast cells showed a complete PAS negativity.

Peroxidase Reaction

ALL and Peroxidase

ALL blast cells were peroxidase-negative.

AGL and Peroxidase

Peroxidase activity was seen in all cases of AGL with azurophilic granules (or Auer rods).

However, it is clear that myeloperoxidase positivity may be seen in the cytoplasm of cells without granules. A great variation of blast cells without azure granules may be seen in AGL; some of them may have myeloperoxidase activity whereas others have none.

However, there were more peroxidase-positive blast cells than cells with azurophilic granules (or Auer rods). The peroxidase reaction is therefore a more sensitive test than the identification of azurophilic granules in diagnosing the myeloid origin of acute leukemia.

The peroxidase reaction, however, is usually of no practical importance, because azurophilic granules are almost always present and suffice for the diagnosis of AGL. There are a few cases where the differential diagnosis of AGL and ALL may be difficult because of absence or the scarcity of azurophilic granules.

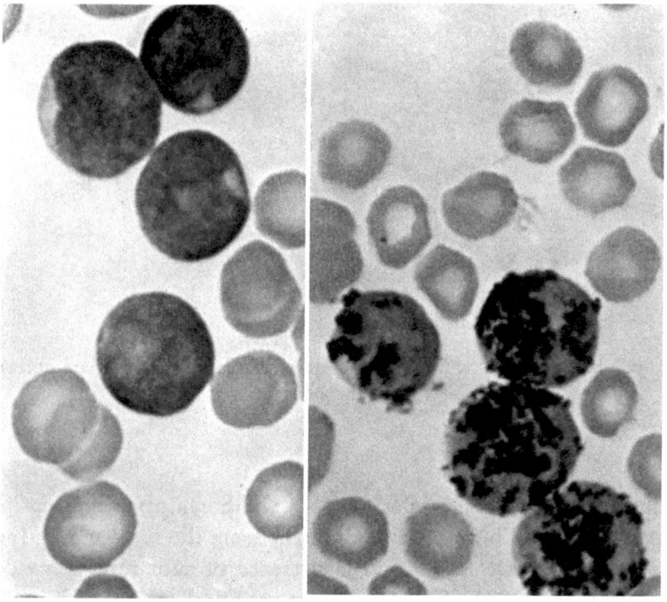

a b

Fig. 3 a and b. Acute granulocytic leukemia, pseudo lymphoblastic pattern. a May-Grunwald-Giemsa preparation — Note the complete agranularity of the blast cells, b Peroxidase reaction in the same patient — Heavy positivity in all the blast cells

In these cases the blast cells may look like myeloblasts without granules, but Auer rods or a few granules, can be found after a careful search.

The striking peroxidase positivity of the majority of the cells in these cases made the diagnosis of AGL easier and more certain. In other cases, the blast cells may look exactly like lymphoblasts of ALL (see Fig. 3) and be completely devoid of Auer rods and azurophilic granules. In these cases, the peroxidase positivity was very obvious in almost all of the blast cells (Fig. 3). This pseudolymphoblastic AGL was not frequent. We think that peroxidase reactivity is sometimes useful.

In relation to this problem, we saw four other cases which we have called ALL because of the cytological and cytochemical features of the cells. However, in a small number of cells, we were able to see myeloperoxidase activity (between 1 and 2% of the blast cells — Fig. 4 —). These positive peroxidase cells were quite different from

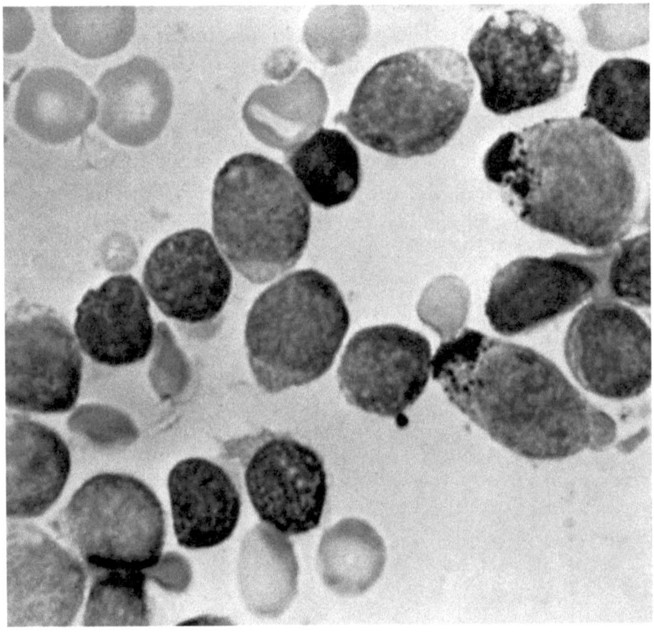

Fig. 4. Acute lymphoblastic leukemia — Peroxidase reaction — Peroxidase activity in 1% to 2% of the blast cells

the few "remaining normal" granulocytic cells which can often be seen in ALL bone marrow. They were small blast cells no different from the surrounding lymphoblasts, except for their peroxidase activity. The presence of such rare peroxidase-positive cells in the peripheral blood of these patients was perhaps an additional reason to suspect that this disease belonged to the myeloid series. This finding is in agreement with BESSIS' electron-microscope observations [3] and may be evidence of a link between pseudo-lymphoblastic AGL with strong myeloperoxidase activity and some of the true "ALL" forms where no peroxidase activity is seen.

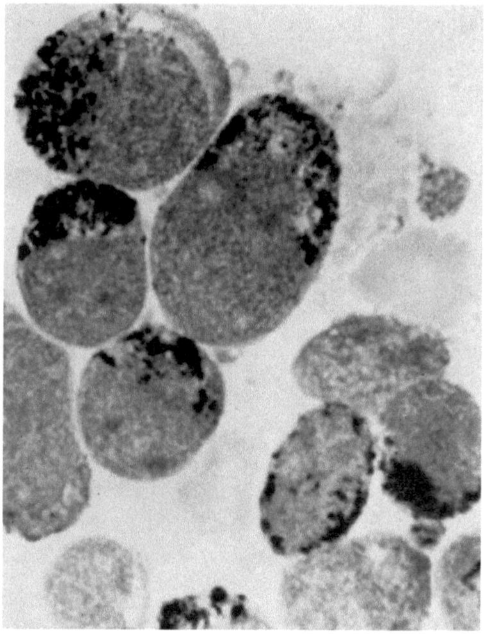

Fig. 5. Acute granulocytic leukemia — Normal peroxidase activity

Peroxidase and Acute Promyelocytic Leukemia

We studied 33 acute promyelocytic leukemias in our series of 921 patients and performed the myeloperoxidase reaction in all 33 cases [7, 8, 21]. The results were very similar. All the blast cells had a very strong positivity completely overlapping the cytoplasm and very often rendering the nucleus invisible. Such a strong peroxidase reaction was never seen in other granulocytic leukemias; it was a help in borderline cases where the granules were thin, reddish and not well defined.

Peroxidase and Acute Monocytic Leukemia

Peroxidase activity varied widely in these cases. In five cases all or nearly all the cells were completely negative; in the others, the positive peroxidase pattern was different from the myeloblastic pattern: a discrete scattered granular positivity was seen on the whole surface of the cell (Fig. 7). When this positivity existed, it was helpful in the diagnosis.

Naphthol AS-D Chloroacetate Esterase Activity

The results with this technique were very similar to those given by peroxidase reaction. However, the monocytic cells were always negative with this reaction, and in the granulocytic series, the reaction was less sensitive than the peroxidase reaction. We have compared these two techniques in 40 acute leukemias [6]. The naphthol AS-D chloroacetate esterase activity was always negative in acute monocytic leukemia

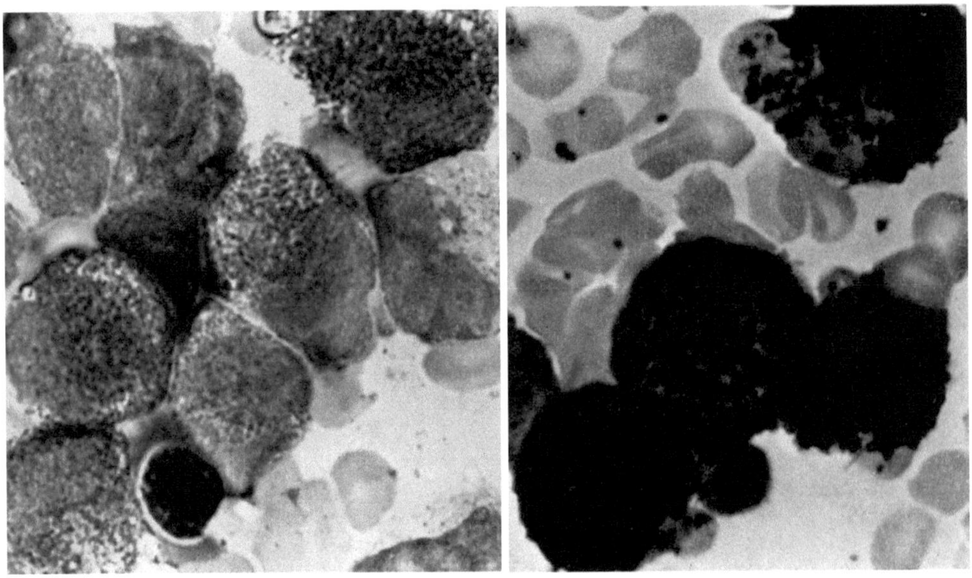

a b

Fig. 6 a and b. Acute promyelocytic leukemia. a MGG preparation, b Peroxidase reaction — very strong positivity, completely overlapping the cytoplasm

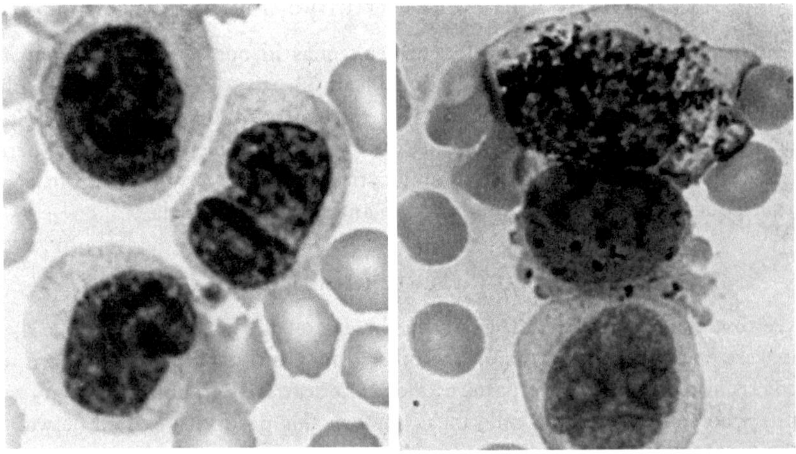

a b

Fig. 7 a and b. Acute monocytic leukemia. a MGG preparation, b Peroxidase reaction — Peroxidase activity ranging from negativity to a discrete scattered granular positivity

(5 cases) and in ALL (12 cases). In AGL and acute myelomonocytic leukemia, it was always less reliable for diagnosis than the peroxidase reaction. In six cases of promyelocytic leukemia, it was strongly positive but slightly less so than peroxidase.

Naphthol AS-D Acetate Esterase Activity

This technique enabled us to distinguish clearly between cases of acute monocytic leukemia and acute leukemias of other cellular types. In acute monocytic leukemia, the majority of the blastic cells possessed a high esterase activity yet this esterase activity was inhibited by sodium fluoride [5].

In a previously reported series of 40 patients we showed [6, 7] that only acute leukemia of the monocytic type possess this pattern of reactivity. Since 1970, we have

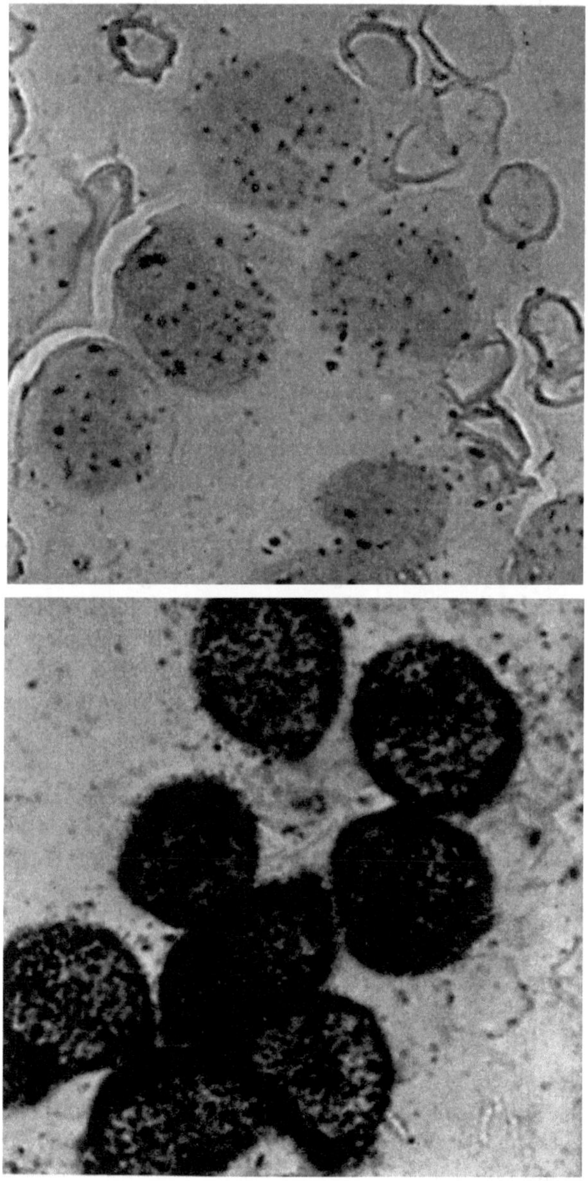

a b

Fig. 8 a and b. Acute monocytic leukemia. a Naphthol AS-D acetate esterase reaction: high esterase activity in all the blast cells, b N AS-D acetate reaction, inhibited by sodium fluoride, in the same patient applied this technique in all the cases where monocytic leukemia was suspected and we have now seen 11 cases of these types of leukemia. In 14 cases, we suspected monocytic leukemia but in 3 cases strong peroxidase activity of the myeloblastic type and the absence of esterase monocytic activity forced us to diagnose AGL.

Discussion

Opinions differ on the practical utility of cytochemical techniques in the diagnosis of the acute leukemias. Hayhoe [11] demonstrated the inadequacy of classification based on MGG stains only. Many authors have proposed various methods of staining and scoring [1, 11, 13, 15] so as to enable investigators from different centers to classify blast cells more uniformly than previously. However, a universally accepted cytochemical classification is still lacking. Most therapeutic data on acute leukemia are based on the classical cytological classification [2], which allows a clear distinction only between ALL and the other more differentiated forms.

In the absence of a definitive cytochemical classification, we use cytochemical reactions in order to obtain more accurate subdivision in ALL, AGL, acute promyelocytic and acute monocytic leukemia.

The statistical data provided by numerous publications in this field are of little help in making a precise classification of each new case of acute leukemia. This is why we think that the PAS reactivity is not much help here. We had 24 cases that were completely PAS-negative, 19 cases quite negative, and 11 cases showing a non-specific pattern of fine granular positivity. Yet the cytological patterns of these negative or poorly positive cases are not really different from the positive ones. A "typical" coarse granular PAS positivity is indeed helpful but it does not occur often enough to be used as a basic criterion for classification.

Our observations on the relative frequency of negativity of PAS reaction in ALL are not unique. Löffler [15] found 10 negative cases among 21 adult cases, and 2 negative cases among 32 childhood cases of ALL; Huhn *et al.* [12] found 3 negative cases out of 9 with ALL; Bennet *et al.* [1] found 7 negative cases out of 28 with ALL. Other authors have mentioned negative cases without giving the specific figure [13, 18]. Hayhoe *et al.* [9], on the contrary, think that in most cases many of the blast cells give a positive reaction.

On attempting to correlate PAS reactivity in ALL with the cytological sub-classification, we did not find any obvious correlation, although the "typical" coarse granule positivity is three times less frequent in sub-class 1 (Mathé's prolymphoblastic type) and this sub-class contains five times more adults. However, the value of this finding depends on the accuracy of the cytological sub-classification (Table 4). As a concluding remark regarding the ALL group, we believe, that the most reliable cytochemical reaction for diagnosis is the peroxidase negativity.

Indeed we think there is the greatest difficult in distinguishing ALL from some cases of AGL where the microblasts show no granulation. The systematic use of the peroxidase reaction in all cases of acute leukemia which are not obviously myeloblastic is very helpful. The use of the peroxidase reaction is of no practical value in cases of acute leukemia with obvious azurophilic granules (or Auer rods).

The Naphthol AS-D chloroacetate esterase reaction is less sensitive than the peroxidase reaction and is not practical.

The Naphthol AS-D acetate esterase, followed by monocytic specific esterase inhibition by sodium fluoride, is a very reliable reaction for the diagnosis of acute monocytic leukemia. However, we do not recommend its systematic use. It should be reserved for cases where the cytology suggests acute monocytic leukemia. Daniel *et al.* [4] showed that, in other cases, this reaction is not of great help. On the other hand, in the field of myelomonocytic leukemias the NAF esterase inhibition is of great help in permitting a clear-cut separation between these cases and the acute monocytic leukemias in which all the cells have a high monocytic esterase activity in the blood and in the bone marrow.

References

1. Bennet, J. M., Dutcher, T. F.: The cytochemistry of acute leukemia observations on glycogen and neutral fat in bone marrow aspirates. Blood **33**, 341 (1969).
2. Bernard, J., Jacquillat, C., Weil, M.: Treatment of acute leukemias. Sem. Hemat. **9**, 181 (1972).
3. Bessis, M., Maigne, J.: Le diagnostic des variétés de leucémies aiguës par la réaction des péroxydases au microscope électronique. Son intérêt et ses limites. Rev. Europ. clin. biol. **15**, 691 (1970).
4. Daniel, M. T., Flandrin, G., Lejeune, F., Liso, P., Lortholary, P. I.: Les estérases spécifiques monocytaires. Utilisation dans la classification des leucémies aiguës. Nouv. Rev. franç. Hémat. **11**, 233 (1971).
5. Fischer, R., Schmalzl, F.: Über die Hemmbarkeit der Esterase Aktivität in Blutmonocyten durch Natriumfluorid. Klin. Wschr. **42**, 751 (1964).
6. Flandrin, G., Daniel, M. T., Blanchet, P., Briere, J., Bernard, J. II: La leucémie aiguë monocytaire. Situation clinique et pronostique à la lumière des techniques de détermination des estérases spécifiques. Nouv. Rev. franç. Hémat. **11**, 241 (1971).
7. Flandrin, G., Daniel, M. T.: Classification morphologique des leucémies aiguës. Actual. Hémat. **4**, 166 (1969).
8. Flandrin, G., Fourcade, M., Daniel, M. T.: Etude cytologique des leucémies aiguës promyélocytaires. Actual. Hémat. **6**, 14 (1972).
9. Hayhoe, F. G., Cawley, J. C.: Acute leukemia: cellular morphology, cytochemistry and fine structure. Clin. haemat. **1**, 49 (1972).
10. Hayhoe, F. G., Flemans, R. J.: An atlas of haematological cytology. London: Wolfe Medical Books (1969).
11. Hayhoe, F. G., Quaglino, D., Doll, R.: The cytology and cytochemistry of acute leukemia. A study of 140 cases. London: HMSO (1964).
12. Huhn, D., Schmalzl, F.: Licht- und elektronenmikroskopische Cytochemie der unreifzelligen Leukämien. Klin. Wschr. **50**, 423 (1972).
13. Leinonen, F. A.: Cytochemical studies of acute leukemia. Acta Haemat. (Basel) **43**, 219 (1970).
14. Löffler, H.: Zytochemischer Nachweis von unspezifischer Esterase in Ausstrichen. Klin. Wschr. **39**, 1220 (1961).
15. Löffler, H.: Zytochemische Klassifizierung der akuten Leucosen. Chemo- und Immunotherapie der Leukosen und malignen Lymphome, p. 120. Wien: Bohmann-Verlag 1969.
16. Mathé, G., Pouillart, P., Sterescu, Marina, Amiel, J. L., Schwarzenberg, G., Schneider, M., Hayat, M., De Vassal, Françoise, Jasmin, C., Lafleur, M.: Subdivision of classical varieties of acute leukemia. Correlation with prognosis and cure expectancy. Europ. J. clin. biol. Res. **16**, 554 (1971).
17. Mathé, G., Seman, G.: Aspects histologiques et cytologiques des leucémies et hématosarcomes. Paris: Maloine, édit. 1963.

18. Melnick, P. J.: Histochemical enzymology of leukaemic cells. Pathology of leukaemia ch. 4, p. 125. Ed.: G. D. Amromin. New York: Hoeber 1968.
19. Moloney, W. C., McPherson, K., Fliegelman, L.: Esterase activity in leukocytes demonstrated by the use of naphthol AS-D chloroacetate substrate. J. Histochem. Cytochem. **8**, 200 (1960).
20. Rozenszajn, L., Leibovich, M., Shoham, D., Epstein, J.: The esterase activity in megaloblasts, leukaemic and normal haematopoietic cells. Brit. J. Haemat. **14**, 605 (1968).
21. Weil, M., Jacquillat, C., Flandrin, G., Boiron, M., Bernard, J.: Clinical and therapeutical studies in acute promyelocytic leukemia. Proc. Amer. Ass. Cancer Res. **13**, 49 (1972).

Indications and Limits of Cytochemistry in Acute Leukemia

H. Löffler

Medizinische Kliniken und Polikliniken der Justus-Liebig Universität, Gießen/Germany

Progress in the therapy of acute leukemia has led to the conclusion that there are at least two groups of acute leukemias differing with respect to the effect of therapy and prognosis. One group is usually referred to as acute lymphatic or lymphoblastic leukemia; the other group includes the granulocytic, myelomonocytic and monocytic varieties as well as erythremic myelosis.

These findings have stimulated attempts to find new classifications for acute leukemias because classification based only on Giemsa staining techniques sometimes appeared arbitrary or uncertain [4, 5, 7, 12].

A year ago a new classification, based upon conventional staining techniques, was proposed by Mathé *et al.* "in order to try to establish a correlation between prognosis and cytological varieties".

The purpose of our own investigations, parts of which have been published earlier [8, 9], was to find out if a classification based only on cytochemical methods could form a basis for therapy.

The following methods have been of practical value in our laboratory and in the hands of other investigators: reactions for the demonstration of peroxidase, alkaline and acid phosphatase, esterase, β-glucuronidase, Sudan black B, and periodic acid Schiff (PAS) reactions. They were applied in several combinations to all cases of acute leukemia in our clinic or those sent to me (so far 380 cases).

It has been our experience that four reactions are sufficient for practical use: peroxidase, esterase (substrates α-naphthyl acetate and Naphthol AS-D chloroacetate) and PAS (Figs. 1 and 2). For evaluation it is necessary to qualify the PAS pattern and to quantify esterase and peroxidase reactions because in the case of naphthyl acetate esterase reaction only a strong activity (grades 3 and 4 in our definition) can be used as a marker reaction. It is not sufficient to define a case of leukemia as PAS-positive or esterase-positive. Additional information may be obtained in special cases by the application of the β-glucuronidase, acid phosphatase reactions and the iron staining techniques.

Cytochemical marker reactions which lead to the demonstration of characteristic patterns in the various cell types involved in the acute leukemias have been used to distinguish the different types. This analysis showed that the cases were separable into five groups (with the exception of erythremic myelosis and rare varieties, which will be discussed later).

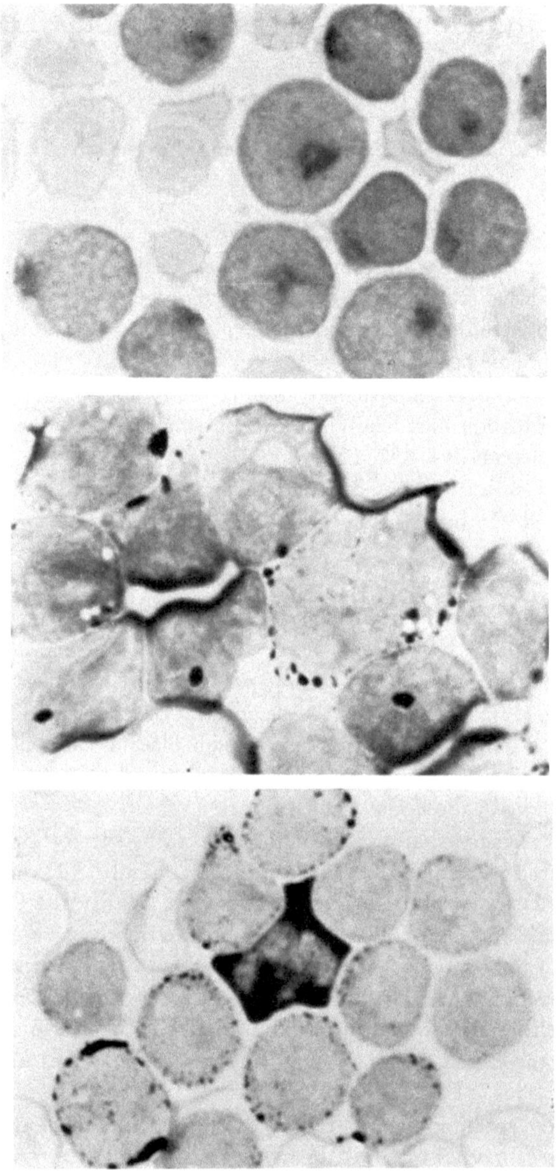

a b c

Fig. 1. a and b. PAS reaction. All the primitive cells are positive with granules and blocks. There is no diffuse staining, c Acid phosphatase reaction. The primitive cells show a distinct paranuclear positivity. Prognosis seems to be poorer in these patients than in the other patients with PAS-type leukemia. ×100

The classification based upon these investigations is shown in Table 1.

There was a limited number of patients who had not been treated before and who had been classified according to the parameters given above. We tried to find out in a retrospective study[1] whether there is a correlation between the effect of therapy, median survival and the types of our classification.

---

1 In cooperation with Dr. PRALLE (Gießen), Dr. FISCHER and Dr. ROUX (I. Med. Univ.-Klinik Mainz) and Dr. LÜCK (Univ.-Kinderklinik Gießen).

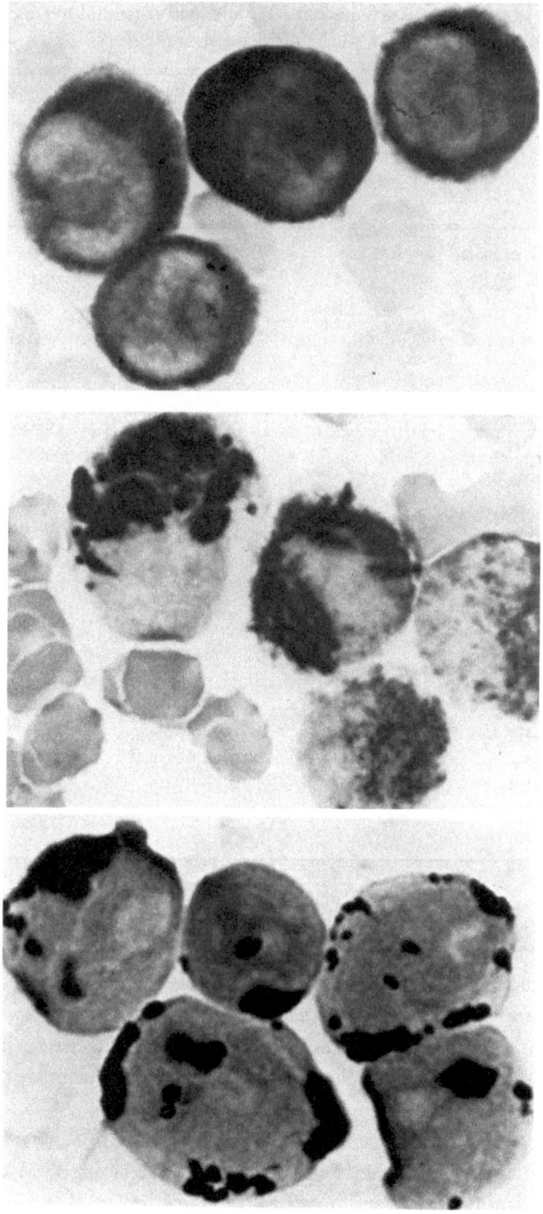

Fig. 2. a Peroxidase reaction. Five primitive cells showing coarse granular positivity, b Naphthol AS-D chloroacetate esterase. Two primitive cells with strongly positive Auer rods and bodies, two cells with positive azurophilic granules, c α-Naphthylacetate esterase. Four primitive cells showing intense positivity (rating 4). Esterase type leukemia. ×1400

Table 2 shows the results of this study. In spite of the rather limited number of patients, the conclusion may be drawn that the group of acute leukemias which fulfills the criteria of PAS type in children and adults is inclined to respond favorably to therapy.

This PAS-type group includes some cases (two in our series who did not respond to therapy with a complete remission) which show a distinct positive acid phosphatase

Table 1. Cytochemical classification of acute leukemias. The conventional terms (left side) are put in relation to the cytochemical ones (right side)

Type of leukemia (Cytological classification)	Cytochemical methods for differentiation			Cytochemical classification
	PAS	Peroxidase % positive	Naphthylacetate esterase % grades 3+4	
Myeloblastic	negative, faint diffuse, rare granules	1—64	< 25	Peroxidase type 1 and 2
Promyelocytic	in most cases moderate diffuse	$\geqq 65$	< 25	Peroxidase type 3
Myelo-monocytic	faint diffuse and moderate granular or negative	in most cases > 50	25—49	Peroxidase — esterase type
Monocytic		in most cases < 25	$\geqq 50$	Esterase type
Undifferentiated	0	0	0	Undifferentiated
Lymphoblastic	granules and blocks, no diffuse reaction	0	0	PAS type
Erythremic myelosis (erythroblasts)	in most cases intense positivity (diffuse or granular)	0	stronger positivity than in normal erythroblasts	

reaction within a small paranuclear area (Fig. 1 c). From the observation that early erythroblasts in normal marrow show the same acid phosphatase pattern and some other details, Drescher and Leder considered these cases to be extremely immature erythremias. I do not think that the information obtained is sufficient to justify this conclusion; nevertheless, prognosis in this small group of patients seems poorer than in the other PAS-type cases.

Since most of the cases classified as PAS-type leukemias fulfill the criteria of "acute lymphoblastic leukemia", our results support the conclusions of Mathé *et al.* that there are differences among the cases classified as acute lymphoblastic leukemia. It would be stimulating to learn more about these cases.

Some of the more rare varieties of acute leukemia are not included in the classification given above. They are discussed briefly. Basophilic leukemia, according to various authors, is a variant of granulocytic leukemia; it can easily be identified by the metachromatic reaction of its granules after toluidine blue or other appropriate staining. Another variant of granulocytic leukemia is eosinophilic leukemia, the existence of which is still doubted by some authors. In 1969 we published our findings in three cases which otherwise showed all the signs and the course of

Table 2. Results of treatment correlated with the cytochemically classified leukemia types in adults. All patients treated for more than 7 days are included

Type	Number of patients	C. R.	Median * survival (days)	Alive
PAS adults	14	86% (12/14)	> 417	2 (June 1972)
PAS children	20	90% (18/20)	> 399	17 (28. 4. 71)
Undifferentiated	4	1/4	151	∅
Peroxidase	26	23% (6/26)	185	∅
Esterase + Perox.-Est.	13	23% (3/13)	135	∅
All "Not-PAS-Type"	43	23% (10/43)	167	∅

* From diagnosis.

Table 3. Typical cytochemical reactions in eosinophilic and basophilic leukemia

Type of leukemia	Typical reactions
Eosinophilic	Naphthol AS-D chloroacetate esterase reaction positive in the eosinophilic granules, acid phosphatase and PAS reactions much stronger than in normal eosinophils
Basophilic	Metachromatic granules after toluidine blue staining

acute leukemia. They were characterized by a positive Naphthol AS-D chloroacetate reaction of the eosinophilic granules — a reaction which has not been obtained in eosinophils in other diseases, or in normal blood and marrow. This observation has been confirmed by Leder (1 case), Schaefer *et al.* (1 case) and in two further cases of our own material. Furthermore in the eosinophils of these patients a heavy PAS positivity and a raised acid phosphatase activity has been found (Table 3).

A highly characteristic cytochemical pattern may be obtained in acute erythremias (erythremic myelosis) and in the erythroblasts of erythroleukemia. The pathological erythroblasts usually show heavy PAS positivity, generally granular in early erythroblasts and diffuse in later ones. In thalassemia major, the only disease which may present with comparable amounts of PAS positivity, the PAS reaction is confined to polychromatophilic and to oxyphilic normoblasts, and it is found in granular form [1, 3]. Additional information may be obtained by applying the naphthyl acetate esterase technique and the iron stain.

Table 4 compares cytochemical findings in erythroblastic disorders.

To sum up: in general, cytochemical techniques proved helpful in classifying and/or identifying acute or immature leukemias.

With rare exceptions, diagnosis depends on conventional cytological staining techniques and clinical findings.

Table 4. Cytochemical reactions of erythroblasts in erythroblastic disorders

	PAS	Iron (Sideroblasts)	Nonspecific esterase
Erythremic myelosis	+++ (diffuse and granular)	+−++ ring sideroblasts rare	++
Thalassemia major	+−++ (granular in mature forms)	+−++	+
Megaloblastic anemias	0	+−++ no ring sideroblasts	+++
Sideroachrestic anemias	(+)	+++ many ring sideroblasts	+

References

1. Astaldi, G., Rondanelli, E. G., Bernadelli, E., Strosselli, E.: An abnormal substance present in the erythroblasts of thalassaemia major. Cytochemical investigations. Acta haemat. (Basel) **12**, 145 (1954).
2. Drescher, J., Leder, L.-D.: Zur Frage der akuten extrem unreifzelligen Erythraemie. Z. Kinderheilk. **108**, 117 (1970).
3. Fessas, Ph., Papayannopoulou, Th.: Cytochemical observations on β-thalassaemia. Acta haemat. (Basel) **34**, 1 (1965).
4. Hayhoe, F. G. J., Quaglino, D., Doll, R.: The cytology and cytochemistry of acute leukaemias. A study of 140 cases. London: HMSO 1964.
5. Hermansky, F.: La valeur de quelques methodes cytochimiques dans la classification des leucoses immatures et atypiques. Nouv. Rev. franç. Hémat. **8**, 239 (1968).
6. Leder, L.-D.: Akute myelo-monocytäre Leukämie mit atypischen Naphthol-AS-D-Chloracetat-Esterase-positiven Eosinophilen. Acta haemat. (Basel) **44**, 52 (1970).
7. Löffler, H.: Hinweise zur Unterscheidung unreifzelliger Leukämien mit zytochemischen Methoden. Dtsch. med. Wschr. **88**, 1531 (1963).
8. Löffler, H.: Eine Klassifizierung als Grundlage der Behandlung unreifzelliger Leukosen. Hämatologie und Bluttransfusion, vol. 8, p. 105. H. Heimpel, L. Heilmeyer, München: J. F. Lehmann 1969.
9. Löffler, H.: Zytochemische Klassifizierung der akuten Leukosen. Chemo- und Immunotherapie der Leukosen und malignen Lymphome, p. 120. Ed.: A. Stacher. Wien: Bohmann 1969.
10. Mathé, G., Pouillart, P., Sterescu, M., Amiel, J. L., Schwarzenberg, L., Schneider, M., Hayat, M., De Vassal, F., Jasmin, C., Lafleur, M.: Subdivision of classical varieties of acute leukaemia. Correlation with prognosis and cure expectancy. Europ. J. clin. biol. Res. **16**, 554 (1971).
11. Schaefer, H. E., Hellriegel, K. P., Hennekeuser, H. H., Hübner, G., Zach, J., Fischer, R.: Unreifzellige Leukose mit Chloroacetat-Esterase positiver Eosinophile („Eosinophilenleukämie"). 15. Dtsch. Hämatologen-Kongr. 1971, Springer, in press.
12. Schmalzl, F., Braunsteiner, H.: The application of cytochemical methods to the study of acute leukaemia. Acta haemat. (Basel) **45**, 209 (1971).

Cytologic Diagnosis of Leukemias by Electron Microscopy

M. Bessis

Institut de Pathologie Cellulaire, Hôpital de Bicêtre, Université de Paris, Paris/France

Many details of cellular organelles are revealed by the electron microscope. This fact aroused the hope that examination of the ultrastructure of white cells could be a significant aid in the diagnosis of leukemias. It is the purpose of this communication to indicate the limited extent to which this hope has been realized and to describe certain pathophysiologic features of leukemic cells which may explain why electron microscopy is only occasionally of diagnostic value.

I. Identifying a Cell as Leukemic

First of all, there is to day (1972) no *single* morphologic marker which can identify a white blood cell as leukemic. There are indeed, certain morphologic features which are suggestive of malignancy, particularly when these features are pronounced or when more than one of them is present in a clone of cells, but some of these characteristics can be studied as well, or better, with the light microscope. These features may be grouped under two headings:

1. anarchy of maturation of the different cell organelles;
2. pathology of cell organelles.

1. Divergence of nuclear and cytoplasmic maturation can often be distinguished as readily by light microscopy as by electron microscopy. However, since the ultrastructure of organelles and granules can only be seen with the electron microscope, certain features of asynchrony, particularly anarchy of organelles, can only be distinguished by electron microscopy. For example, leukemic cells may have the pale nucleus of a myeloblast with large nucleoli, associated with the proportions of primary (azurophilic) and secondary (neutrophilic) granules characteristic of normal promyelocytes, myelocytes, or even mature neutrophils. Or take asynchrony in the development of phagocytosis and morphologic maturation: phagocytic ability can be assessed in electron micrographs by ingestion of red cells, when present; often however, the best criterion of phagocytic ability is to add starch particles or killed streptococci to a blood or marrow suspension and examine it after brief incubation in either supravital preparations or stained smears. In general, the phagocytic ability of malignant cells is considered to be less than that of their normal counterparts, but on occasions leukemic promyelocytes and even blast cells may have phagocytic ability, which normally develops only at the late myelocyte stage.

The concept of "maturation anarchy" was suggested (Bessis, 1957, 1968) to explain the loss in leukemic cells of normal sequence and interdependence in the development of such organelles as Golgi bodies, azurophilic and specific granules, ribosomes, mitochondria, etc. This might be, as it were, a failure of the "program"

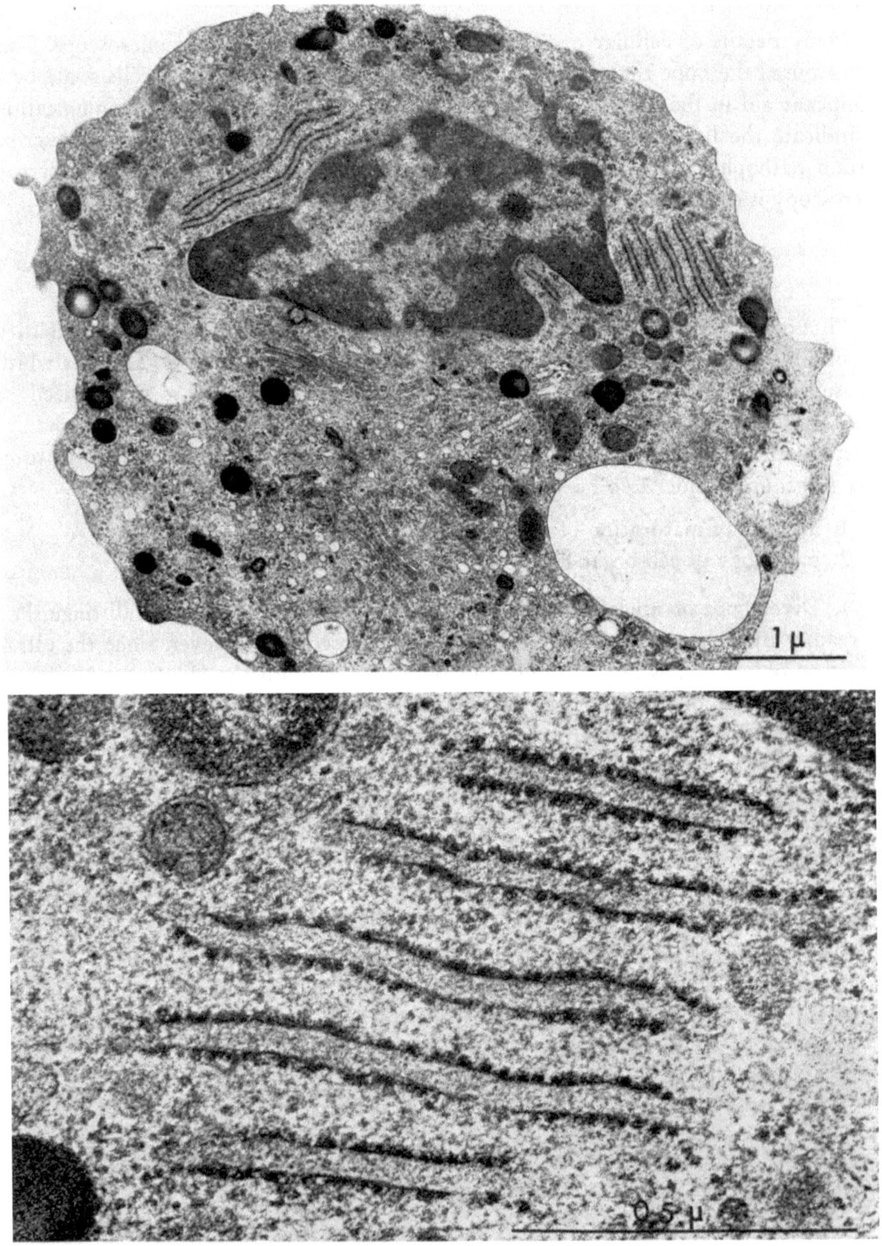

Fig. 1. *Nucleo-cytoplasmic anarchy in a granulocyte.* Persistence of endoplasmic reticulum; absence of secondary granules

for cell maturation. As a consequence, abnormal proportions of individual organelles will appear at unexpected times, perhaps even spatially segregated, resulting in chaotic mixtures. The most disorganized assemblies of organelles seem to be related to chromosomal abnormalities such as hyperdiploidy and others. A general failure of the normal maturation program may be expected to induce frequent pathologic alterations of individual organelles as well. Such anarchy can only be fully appreciated by electron microscopy.

2. Pathologic alterations may affect various organelles: the Golgi body is often larger than normal; the mitochondria may have an unusual number of myelin figures; ribosomes may persist in mature cells attached to a sac of endoplasmic reticulum (Fig. 1). The nucleus, which can occasionally be seen even with the light microscope, to have a bizarre indentation, may form actual pockets that under the electron microscope are seen to contain cytoplasm filled with granules, or one or both centrioles. The number and size of granules may vary abnormally both within the cell and between one cell and another (BESSIS et BRETON-GORIUS, 1969).

The fibrils normally present may form fibrillar bodies. Under the light microscope these bodies appear as pale areas, 1—3 μ in diameter; when seen with the electron microscope, they have an elongated, often curved or even crescent shape, depending upon the angle of the section. These structures are made up of fibrils arranged circularly, or occasionally in whorls. Sometimes azurophilic granules or a few mitochondria can be seen in the center of these structures. Serial sections reveal that these fibrillar bodies generally have an elongated, cylindrical or oval shape. A hypotonic medium, which will considerably change the appearance of the cytoplasm and the ergastoplasmic structures, has no effect on the appearance of the fibrils. Fibrillar bodies are found in 3—10% of myeloblasts, promyelocytes and myelocytes but never in mature cells. They appear to be degenerative forms of the cytoplasmic fibrils that usually encircle the nucleus although they may sometimes be seen in the interior of the nucleus (Fig. 2). They are not specific to granulocytic leukemia cells since they are also seen in monocytic leukemia and, rarely, in the bone marrow of non-leukemic individuals.

Auer bodies are another pathologic alteration of organelles; in this case of preneutrophilic or pre-basophilic granules. They have not been observed other than in acute leukemias or, very rarely, myeloblastic crises of chronic leukemia. Thus they are very useful diagnostically, although we hesitate to say that they may not be found in a non-leukemic disease state (Fig. 3). As noted at the outset, we consider it axiomatic that no single criterion should be used in the present stage of our knowledge to identify a white cell as leukemic.

It is noteworthy that the changes we have described can also be seen in the granulocytic series of so-called refractory, or sideroblastic anemias (BESSIS *et al.*, 1969) which are known to turn into acute leukemias in a number of instances.

II. Identifying Leukemic Cells Line

Electron microscopy may sometimes be useful in identifying the cell line of an acute leukemia when light microscopy fails to do so. Peroxidase positivity in the perinuclear cistern and in the ergastoplasm can occasionally be identified by electron microscopy in myeloblasts which are peroxidase-negative by light microscopy (BESSIS

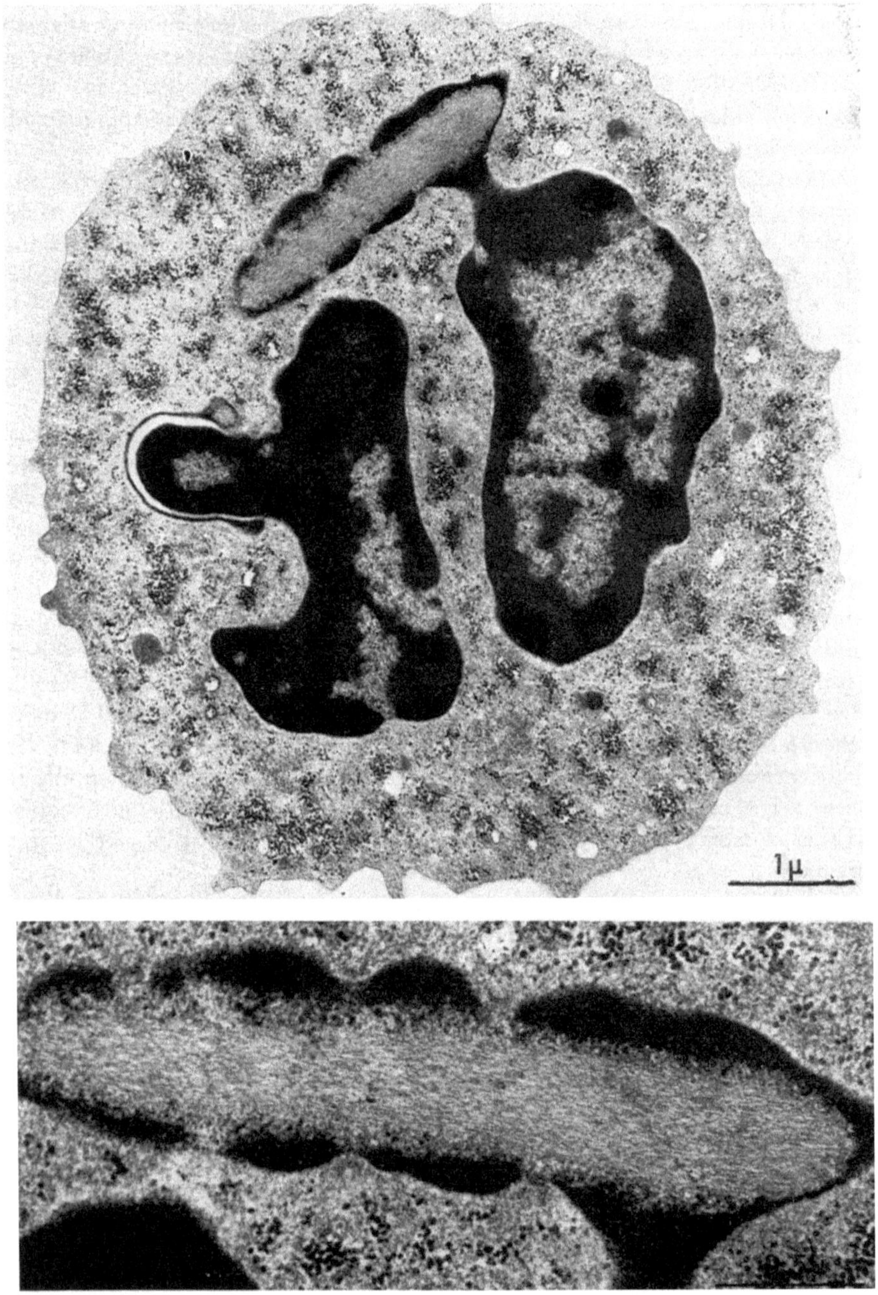

Fig. 2. *Nucleo-cytoplasmic anarchy in a granulocyte.* Absence of granulations. Note the fibrillar body into the nucleus

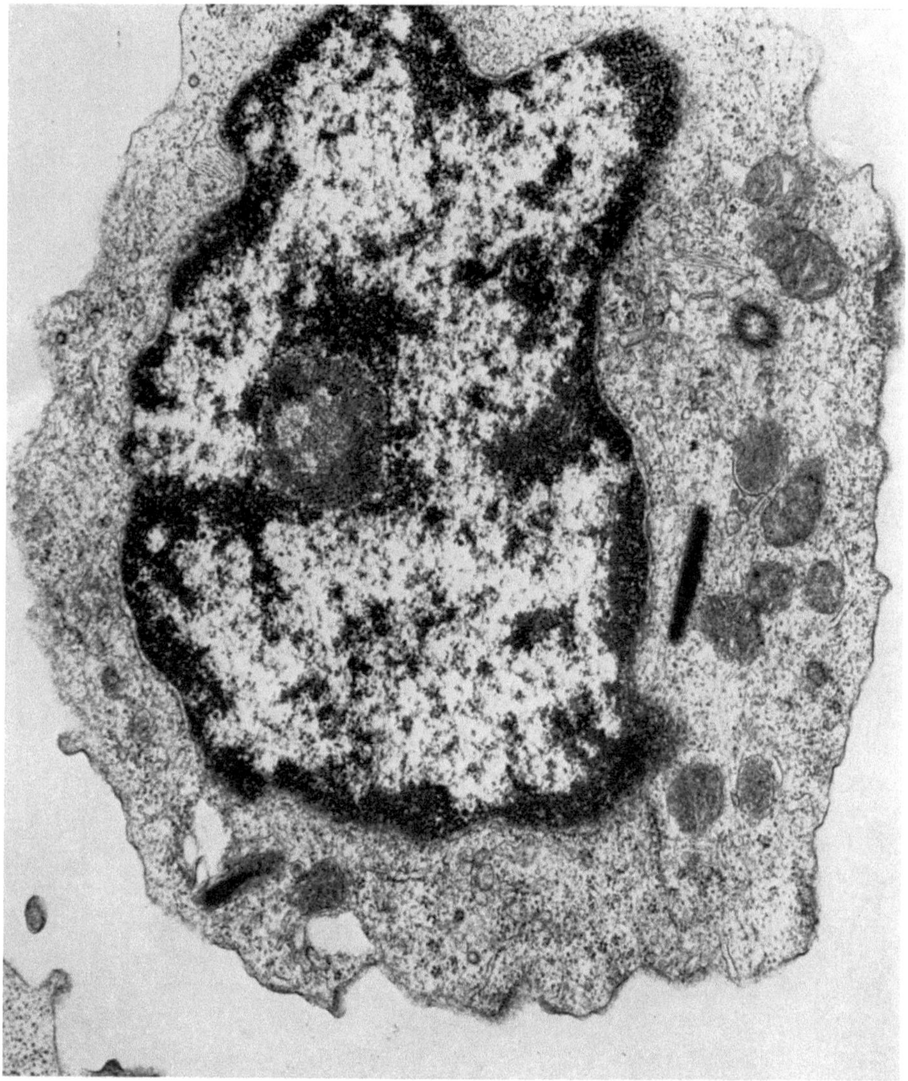

Fig. 3. *Pseudo-monoblastic leukemia.* The electron microscope shows, in some cells, the presence of one micro Auer body. This leukemia was in reality myeloblastic

and MAIGNE, 1970). This may be the only indication of the myeloblastic nature of leukemia (Fig. 4). Monoblastic granules differ sufficiently from azurophilic or neutrophilic granules to identify monoblasts in rare cases. Auer bodies have a special ultrastructure in basophilic myeloblastic leukemia (CECIO *et al.*, 1970). Micro-megacaryocytic leukemias have special characteristics (BRETON-GORIUS *et al.*, 1970).

The more pathologic the alterations of a cell line, the more readily can one conclude that it is leukemic. By the same token however, the more pathologic the cell line, the more difficult it becomes to identify the original cell line and diagnosis of a specific cell line becomes increasingly difficult as the disease progresses.

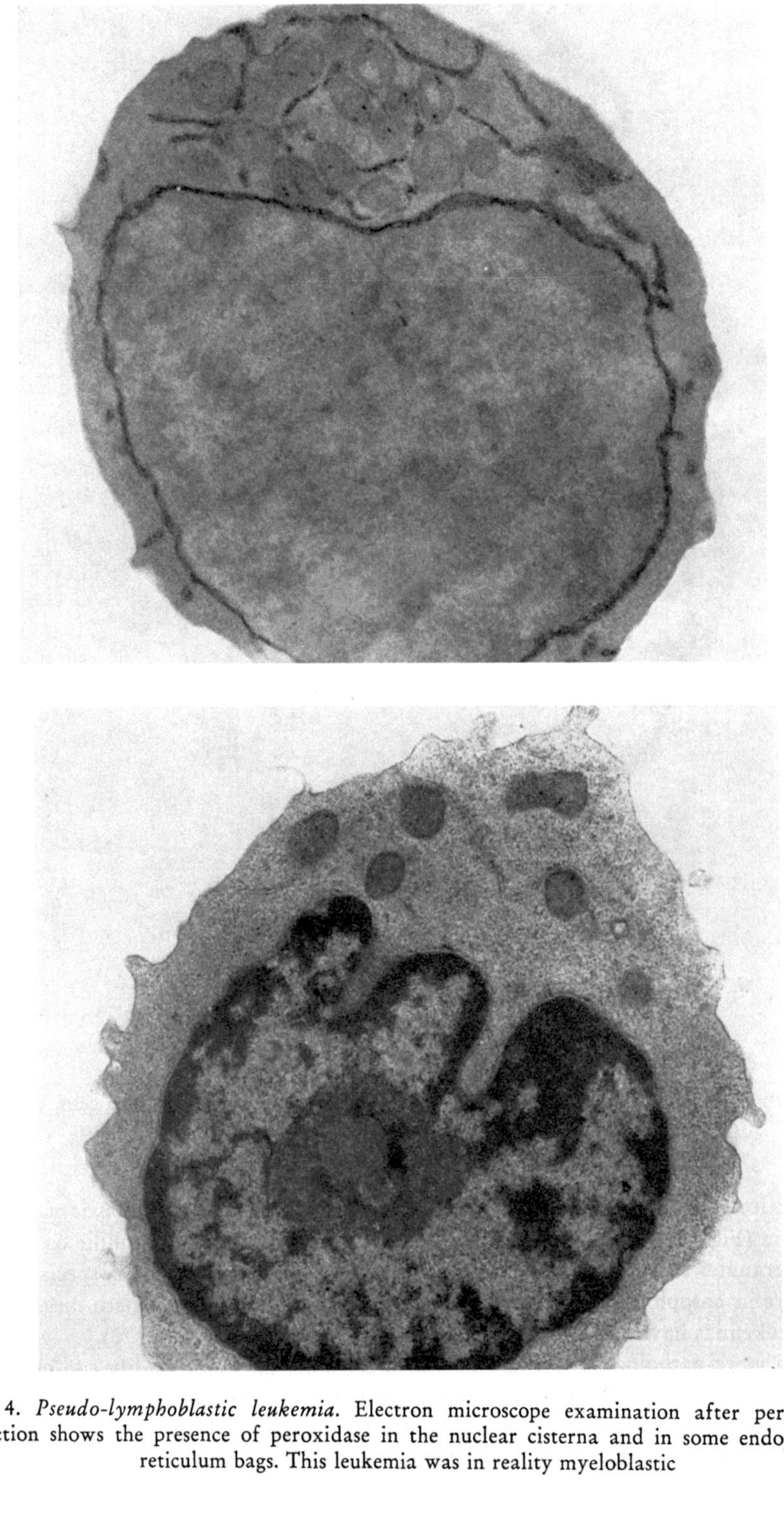

Fig. 4. *Pseudo-lymphoblastic leukemia.* Electron microscope examination after peroxidase reaction shows the presence of peroxidase in the nuclear cisterna and in some endoplasmic reticulum bags. This leukemia was in reality myeloblastic

We have already referred to the anarchy of organelles; this may be so marked that the characteristic features of a given cell line are obscured, or cells may assume the appearance of other cells. For example, myeloblasts that have only a few ribosomes will have a grey cytoplasm when stained with Giemsa and be classified as monoblasts. The pathology of cytoplasmic organelles includes deformities, increases in size, or reductions in volume, which may also make cells take on a misleading morphologic appearance. For example, the nuclei of myeloblasts which are contorted and lobulated may resemble monoblast nuclei. In other cases, the nucleus may be voluminous and correspondingly, the nuclear-cytoplasmic ration will be increased and, if there are no granules, the cell resembles lymphoblasts.

III. Mosaicism and Progression

There are two other processes that occur in malignancies and add to the difficulty: mosaicism and progression. Mosaicism occurs because a number of clones coexist in a leukemic cell population from the beginning, or new clones arise during the development of the disease. It may be impossible to recognize one of these cell clones as belonging to a definite cell line. Some clones, which have a proliferative advantage or acquire it through mutation, proliferate and gain ascendancy over the other clones. In general, such cells are poorly differentiated. "Maturation arrest", of certain leukemic cell clones manifesting at an even earlier stage (BESSIS, 1957); a phenomenon now called "progression". In some cases, progression appears related to the alteration in karyotype that may occur during the evolution of a leukemia (PEDERSEN, 1967, 1969). An increasing simplification of the array of organelles is characteristic of progression and clonal evolution; thus diagnosis of the cell line becomes increasingly difficult as the hallmarks of the differentiated cell are lost.

Finally, chemotherapy can induce pathologic alterations both on the leukemic cell line and on normal cells. For example, in clear-cut cases of lymphoblastic leukemia, vigorous treatment may lead to the development of pathologic myelocytes or promyelocytes, and these may put the initial diagnosis in doubt (BRECHER, 1972). The changes induced by chemotherapy have not yet been studied adequately by electron microscopy. Such a study might help us to separate the entities which can give rise to confusion.

Conclusion

In difficult cases, cytologic diagnosis of the cell line involved can sometimes be established by electron microscopic investigations. However, some unclassifiably cases remain. This is so partly because we still do not have techniques to characterize lymphocytic or monocytic stem cells and partly because leukemic cells are sometimes too "simplified": cells which have lost all capability for specific synthesis cannot be classified by any method of investigation.

References

BESSIS, M.: L'autonomie des cellules leucémiques et des cellules cancéreuses en général. Rev. Hémat. **12**, 142 (1957).

BESSIS, M.: Ultrastructure of normal and leukemic granulocytes. In: Proc. internat. conf. on leukemia-lymphoma, p. 281. Ed.: C. J. D. ZARAFONETIS. Philadelphia: Lea and Febiger 1968.

Bessis, M., Breton-Gorius, J.: Pathologie et asynchronisme de développement des organelles cellulaires au cours des leucémies aiguës granulocytaire. Nouv. Rev. franç. Hémat. **9**, 245 (1969).

Bessis, M., Dreyfus, B., Breton-Gorius, J., Sultan, C.: Etude au microscope électronique de onze cas d'anémies réfractaires avec enzymopathies multiples. Nouv. Rev. franç. Hémat. **9**, 87 (1969).

Bessis, M., Maigne, J.: Le diagnostic des varietés de leucémies aiguës par la réaction des peroxydases au microscope électronique. Son intérêt et ses limites. Rev. Europ. clin. biol. **15**, 691 (1970).

Brecher, G.: Personal Communication 1972.

Breton-Gorius, J., Dreyfus, B., Sultan, C., Basch, A., d'Oliveira, J. G.: Identification of circulating micro-megakaryocytes in a case of refractory anemia: an electron microscopic cytochemical study. Blood **40**, 453 a (1972).

Cecio, A., Dini, E., Quattrin, N.: Prime osservazioni al microscopie elettronico di due casi di leucemia basofila acuta. Boll. Soc. ital. Biol. sper. **46**, 459 (1970).

Pedersen, B.: Evolutionary trends of aneuploid blood culture cell populations during progression and treatment of chronic myelogenous leukaemia. Acta path. microbiol. scand. **69**, 185 (1967).

Pedersen, B.: Cytogenetic Evolution in Chronic Myelogenous Leukaemia. Relation of Chromosomes to Progression and Treatment of the disease. Copenhagen: Munksgaard 1969.

Electron Microscopic Aspects of Cells in the Four Subvarieties of Acute Lymphoid Leukemia

M. Paintrand, D. Dantchev, and G. Mathé

Institut de Cancérologie et d'Immunogénétique*, Hôpital Paul-Brousse**, Villejuif/France

G. Mathé *et al.* [1, 2, 3] have proposed to distinguish, on the basis of the aspects of the leukemic cells on the first bone marrow smear stained by Giemsa, four subvarieties of acute lymphoid leukemia (ALL), called by convention: "prolymphoblastic", "macrolymphoblastic", "microlymphoblastic" and "prolymphocytic".

We have studied, in double-blind fashion, the aspects of the cells of these different subvarieties as seen by electron microscopy (EM).

After gravity sedimentation of the erythrocytes, the leukemic bone marrow specimen was resuspended in the supernatant plasma. Approximately 5×10^6 cells were centrifuged in a conical tube and the pellets were fixed by glutaraldehyde and osmium tetroxide. Ultrathin sections were stained by uranyl acetate and lead citrate.

The four varieties were recognized on EM photographs, and their EM characteristics are given in Table 1 and illustrated by Fig. 1.

One can underline some of them. The "prolymphoblast" presents an irregular nucleus and some ergastoplasmic lamellae. These have been described by Bernhardt and Leplus as "the youngest lymphoblasts" [4]. In contrast, the "macrolymphoblast" has a rounded nucleus and, very rarely, ergastoplasmic lamellae. The "macrolymphoblast" and the "microlymphoblast" differ in size, as do their nucleoli which are large in the "macrolymphoblast" and small in the "microlymphoblast". The "prolymphocyte" appears less undifferentiated. There is a general increase in the contrast within the cell. The chromatin is very concentrated along the nuclear membrane and forms many dense clumps. The nucleolus is seldom visible. The mitochondria are assembled in an invagination of the nucleus.

We can therefore use the electron microscope to confirm the possibility of distinguishing four subvarieties of ALL.

With light microscopy, there is difficulty in distinguishing between the "macrolymphoblast" and "monoblast". As one can see from Table 2 and Fig. 2, the electron microscope allows us to distinguish these cell types very easily.

In conclusion, electron microscopy may assist conventional cytology in the subclassification of acute leukemias when the latter does not permit a precise diagnosis.

---

* INSERM et Association Claude-Bernard.

** 14—16, av. Paul-Vaillant Couturier.

Table 1. Characteristics of cells in the four varieties of acute lymphoid leukemia

		"Prolymphoblast"	"Macrolymphoblast"	"Microlymphoblast"	"Prolymphocyte"
Size (by light microscopy)		16 to 20 μ	12 to 16 μ	8 to 10 μ	10 to 12 μ
	Nucleocytoplasmic ratio	High	High	High	High
Nucleus	Shape	Irregular	Rounded	Rounded	Rounded with invagination
Nucleus	Chromatin	Concentrated along the nuclear membrane	Concentrated along the nuclear membrane Some dense clumps	Concentrated along the nuclear membrane Some dense clumps	Very concentrated along the nuclear membrane Many dense clumps
Nucleus	Nucleolus	Large	Large	Small	Rarely visible
Cytoplasm	Ergastoplasmic lamellae	Some	Very rare	Rare	Very rare
Cytoplasm	Mitochondria	Dispersed around the nucleus	Dispersed around the nucleus	Dispersed around the nucleus	Assembled in an invagination of the nucleus

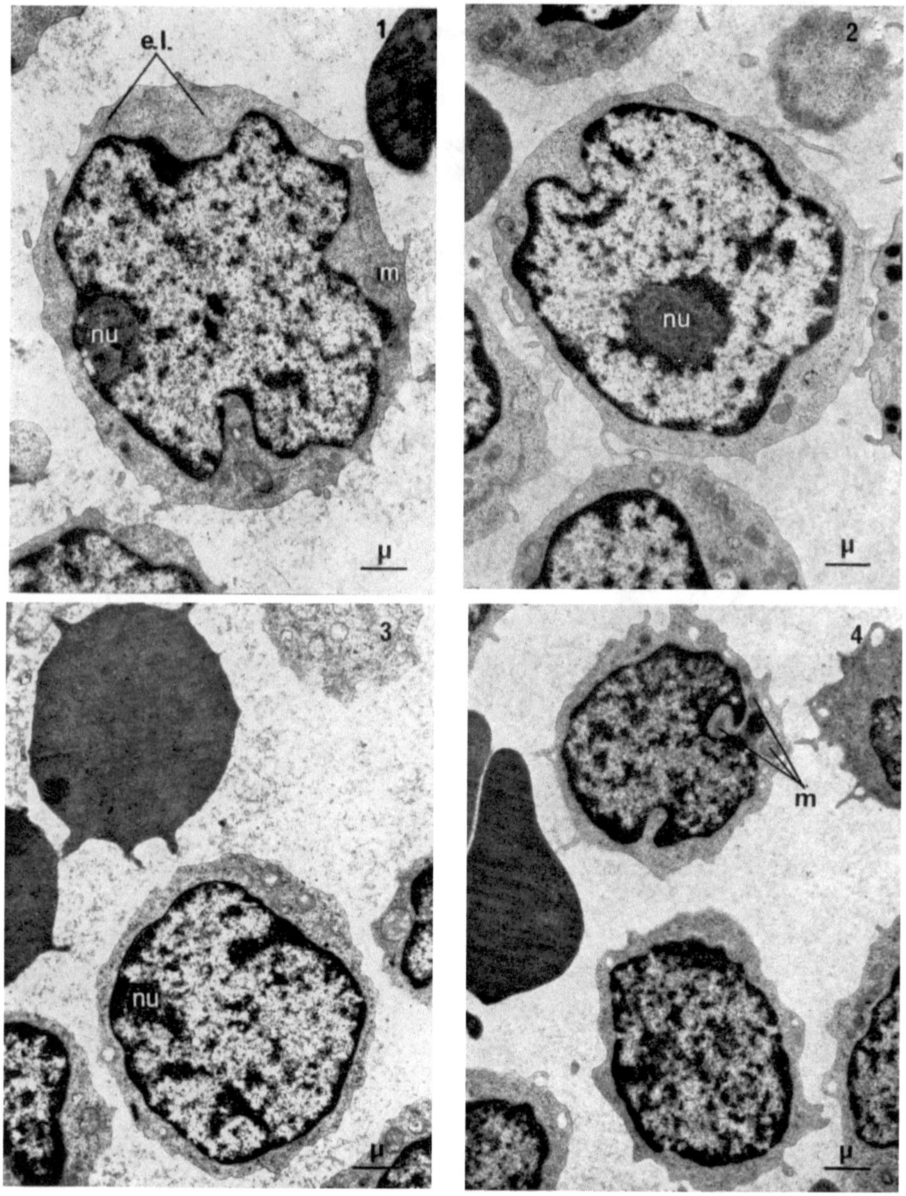

Fig. 1. 1. A cell from a so-called prolymphoblastic subvariety. 2. A cell from a so-called macrolymphoblastic subvariety. 3. A cell from a so-called microlymphoblastic subvariety. 4. Two cells from a so-called prolymphocytic subvariety. (e. l. = ergastoplasmic lamellae; m = mitochondrium; nu. = nucleolus) ×8,000

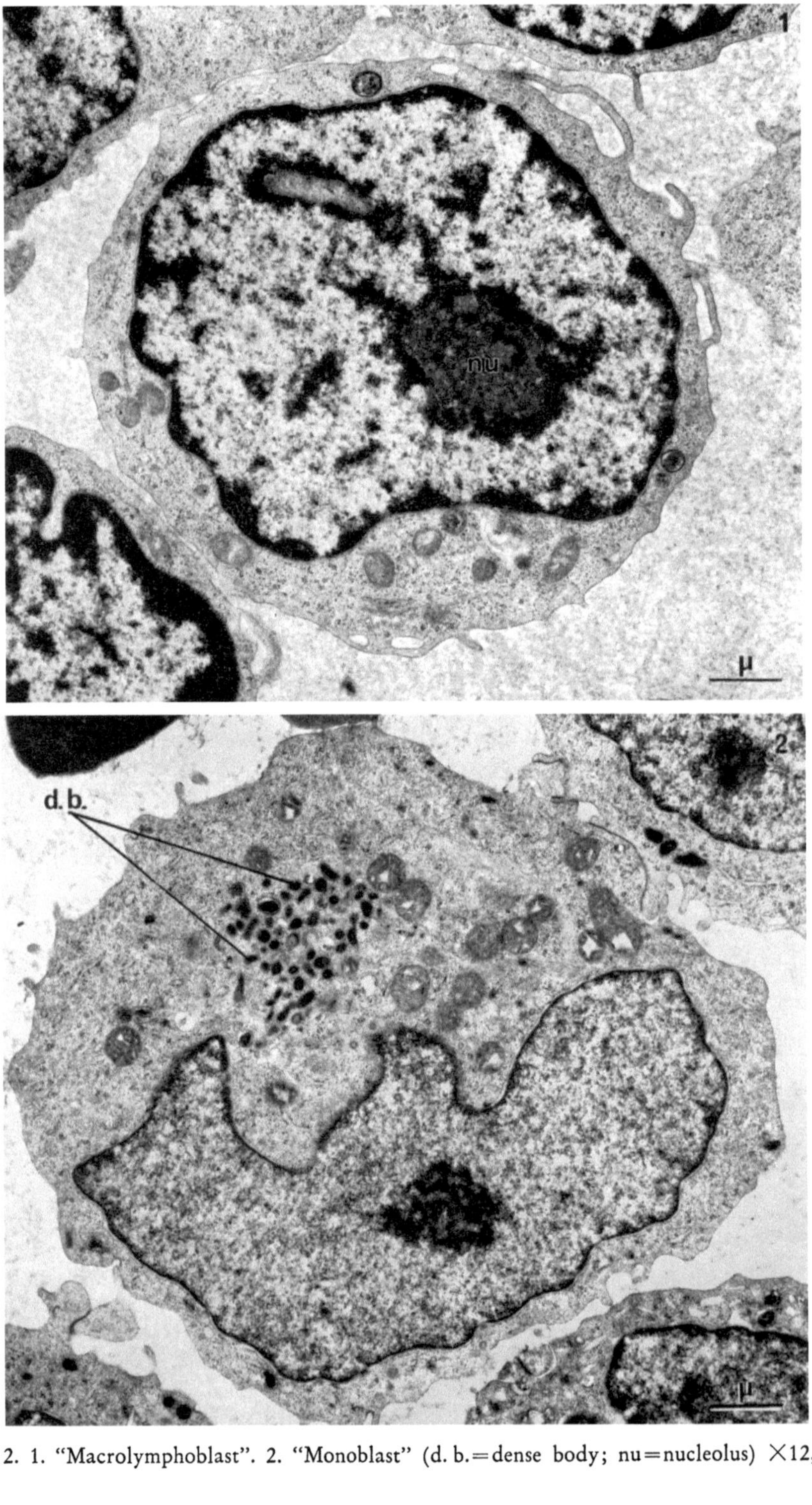

Fig. 2. 1. "Macrolymphoblast". 2. "Monoblast" (d. b.=dense body; nu=nucleolus) ×12,000

Table 2

	"Macrolymphoblast"	"Monoblast"
Nucleocytoplasmic ratio	High	Low
Nucleus	Rounded, one nucleolus	Distorted, several nucleoli
Cytoplasm	Dense bodies: few or none ("Lysosomes")	Dense bodies: many ("Lysosomes")

References

1. Mathé, G., Pouillart, P., Sterescu, M., Amiel, J. L., Schwarzenberg, L., Schneider, M., Hayat, M., De Vassal, F., Jasmin, C., Lafleur, M.: Subdivision of classical varieties of acute leukemia. Correlation with prognosis and cure expectancy. Europ. J. clin. biol. Res. **16**, 554 (1971).
2. Mathé, G., Rappaport, H.: Histological typing of the neoplastic diseases of the haematopoietic and lymphoid tissues. Genève: WHO 1973, in press.
3. Mathé, G., Pouillart, P., Weiner, R., Hayat, M., Sterescu, M., Lafleur, M.: Classification and subclassification of acute leukemias correlated with clinical expression, therapeutic sensitivity and prognosis. p. 6. In: Acute leukemias nomenclature, classification, clinical trials, methodology and actuarial results. Eds.: G. Mathé, P. Pouillart and L. Schwarzenberg. 1 vol. Heidelberg: Springer 1973.
4. Bernhardt, W., Leplus, R.: Fine structure of the normal and malignant human lymph node. Paris: Gauthier-Villars 1964.

Observations on the Kinetics of Acute Lymphoblastic Leukemia in Relation to its Division into Subvarieties

F. GAVOSTO

Division of Hematology, General Medical Clinic, University of Turin, Turin/Italy

A considerable degree of uncertainty has always existed with respect to the histogenetic identification and cytomorphological classification of the acute leukemias. This has led to clashes of opinion and, worse still, to confusion. The main reason is that we still lack reliable descriptive information concerning the stem cells of hematopoietic tissues. Many of their functional properties have been described in some detail: self-maintenance, awareness of the total mass of the population to which they give rise, sensitivity to signals ensuring feedback control over the proliferative and differentiative activities of the pool, the existence of different levels of proliferative potential, and the ability to form clones and develop colonies in irradiated host animals or in soft agar. Yet the paradox remains—their morphological portraits have still to be painted. As far as man is concerned, a question posed half an century ago can still be validly put: Are we dealing with a single population composed of fully omnipotent cells, or are there distinct populations, e.g. precursors of the marrow hematopoietic cells and the lymphocytes?

Since acute leukemia is characterized by relatively homogeneous populations of very young cells, any attempt at classification will obviously be seriously impeded by these uncertainties, and by the absence of any clear understanding of the relationship between stem cells and acute leukemia blasts.

This relationship, in fact, has been established only in kinetic terms. Our own work has shown that the actively proliferating blasts in this disease do not form a self-maintaining population and thus cannot be thought of as stem cells. It would also appear that a class of stem or clonogenic leukemic cells may lie within the population itself. This kinetic approach has enabled more complete and comprehensive growth models to be constructed, based on the presence of three compartments instead of the simple distinction between proliferating and non-proliferating blasts [1]. The existence of leukemic stem cell populations has also been demonstrated in experiments on irradiated animals and agar cultures [10, 11]. Yet, in spite of these advances, if one were to ask a specialist in hematological morphology to point out such cells in a leukemic population, he would not be able to do so.

The objection could, perhaps, be raised that undue emphasis is being given to matters of classification as far as acute leukemia cells are concerned, and that classification and other such dealings in words tend to conceal questions of fact and encourage the obstinate squeezing into categories of things that are not yet known. While valid in general terms, this objection is no longer tenable if we take into consideration that acute leukemia can now be treated in such a way as to modify both its course and prognosis.

A criterion for division and classification can thus be found in the substantially different manner in which subvarieties respond to treatment and are favorably influenced as regards their prognosis. In the case of acute lymphoblastic leukemia (ALL), this criterion has recently been applied [8] and the present paper deals with the kinetic aspects of ALL classification. The specific criteria used to distinguish subvarieties of ALL are differentiation and mean cell size.

The first criterion may rest upon such morphological features as the number and visibility of the nucleoli, the variously fine and reticular appearance of the chromatin, cytoplasmic basophilia, and variations in the nucleus-cytoplasm ratio, perhaps with the aid of cytochemical data (more advanced differentiation may, for example, be accompanied by the appearance of new specific proteins in the cytoplasm).

Cell size is often correlated to the degree of differentiation in the sense that more differentiated cells can be relatively smaller. Yet this general assumption does not hold in the hematological field. In the granulopoietic series, for example, the promyelocyte is larger than the less differentiated myeloblast, while the granular form of the latter is larger than the younger, non-granular form.

More than this, however, recent kinetic studies have made it clear that only limited reliance can be placed on average cell size as a criterion for distinguishing subvarieties of acute leukemia. Cell size is known to vary considerably within any acute leukemia population. Blast diameters may range from 10 to 25 μ, corresponding to areas of 80 to 490 μ^2. Variance *within* a single population, indeed, may often exceed that *between* different cell populations.

Kinetics has both revealed this fact and gone some way to offering a reasonable explanation. Three points in particular are now well known:

1. The size of each actively proliferating cell will depend on the stage of the cell cycle it is in at any given moment. The diameter of blasts in S phase is, on the average, about 12% greater than at the beginning of G_1. This difference has been experimentally determined in the following manner: the mean diameter of the labeled cohort is determined 1 hr after pulse labeling (the labeled blasts are in S or G_2 phase) and then immediately after the first halving of the grains (the labeled cohort is now in G_1 phase). The difference between the two values gives the increase in diameter that the proliferating blasts undergo during the S phase: this is of the order of 12% [1, 4, 5].

2. Not all the cells in a given blast population are actively proliferating at any one moment. Those that form the proliferating compartment, quite apart from their phase-dependent differences in size, are generally larger than those that are out of cycle (G_0) or definitely sterile (Z). This difference in mean size is so well marked that it offers a reliable basis for the calculation of the "growth fraction" of a leukemic population [1, 5].

3. The relative number of large proliferating blasts, and hence the growth fraction, may vary over time in the same patient as a result of the following factors:

a) total number of leukemic cells: when this increases, the number of cells in the proliferating compartment decreases. This inverse relationship is equally applicable to almost all neoplastic populations.

b) growth rate of the cell population: when this increases, as in the case of spontaneous poussées, the relative number of large blasts (and hence the growth fraction) is larger than in the near steady state situation. In other words, recommencement of evolution in leukemia is more the result of an increase in the growth fraction than a shortening of the proliferating cycle time [9].

c) type of treatment employed: for example, if drugs that are active only against cells in cycle are administered, there is a sudden reduction in the number of large blasts and hence in the mean size of the entire population. Later, however, this parameter may again be increased by recruitment into the cycle of resting cells that have survived the attack. Marked fluctuations in the mean size can thus be a result of the type of management employed [2].

These considerations are based on kinetic studies carried out over the last few years. They suggest that a certain degree of caution must be exercised in assessing subvarieties of acute leukemia solely on the basis of mean cell diameter. In themselves, they do not exclude other classification criteria, such as the degree of differentiation; indeed, they support them. In this connection a study has been made of the kinetic features of a series of cases of ALL distinguished as "less" and "more" differentiated. Patients were selected in the relatively steady state and before treatment of any kind had been administered. In the first group (A), cell populations were composed of lymphoblasts with the characteristics of very poorly differentiated cells; in the second (B), a more advanced degree of differentiation could be made out. The morphological criteria already described were employed in making the distinction. Cases in which no clear assignement could be made to either group were excluded.

The labeling index (L. I.) for the whole population and its proliferating compartment, mitotic index (M. I.), growth fraction (G. F.), generation time (T_c) and DNA synthesis time (T_s) are indicated for each group in the Table.

These parameters offer useful indications of the features and proliferative potential of a given population, though it should be borne in mind that a more precise determination of the growth curve (and/or growth rate) would require assessment of the extent of cell loss within the population. It is evident that populations with less differentiated blasts have a higher proliferative potential. This ALL group is closer to acute myeloblastic leukemia and is likewise more frequent in the adult. Where differentiation is more advanced, on the other hand, proliferative activity is much lower. Children are more frequently affected with this last form and a more favorable prognosis is observed for infantile forms.

On the other hand, since the number of blasts in cycle is higher in the first group, it would be expected to be more sensitive to drugs acting solely or primarily on cells in cycle. Yet this relationship, if indeed it exists, must be considered as applicable to nothing more than the start of a chemotherapeutic course. Once the actively proliferating blasts have been destroyed, it is clear from the latest kinetic evidence that there is a recall into cycle of blasts that were quiescent at the moment of chemical attack; moreover, this summons may sometimes occur in a synchronous fashion. The position seems to be that the sensitivity to any particular regimen in a case of acute leukemia, and hence the possibility of remission and its duration, will depend not

Table. Kinetic parameters in two sub-varieties of human acute lymphoblastic leukemia

Variety	Case	L. I. [a]	L. I. p. [b]	M. I. [c]	G. F. [d]	T_C [e]	T_S [f]
A: lymphoblasts with a very low degree of differentiation	I. G.	9.3	15.3	0.15	0.58	104	16
	M. A.	19.9	32.6	0.22	0.61	58	19
	G. A.	12.5	26	0.43	0.48	65	17
	M. P.	9.7	20.6		0.47	77	16
B: lymphoblasts with a more advanced degree of differentiation	M. B.	5.2	20.8	0.10	0.25	78	16
	R. B.	2.4	10.9	0.03	0.22	173	19
	N. L.	5.7	19	0.15	0.30	85	16
	G. O.	5.9	15.9	0.30	0.37	125	21
	R. A.	3.1	10.3	0.30	0.30	155	16

[a] L. I. = labelling index of the whole blast population.
[b] L. I. p. = labelling index of the proliferating blasts.
[c] M. I. = mitotic index.
[d] G. F. = growth fraction (in percent).
[e] T_C = generation time (in hours).
[f] T_S = DNA synthesis time (in hours).

merely on the relative number of cycling blasts but on the intercompartmental flow patterns during the treatment itself. Unfortunately, no clear picture yet exists concerning these cell movements in either the induction or the maintenance stage. This means that kinetic data obtained in particular cases or during various treatment stages cannot be put to wider use. No kinetic explanation is yet to hand for the greater sensitivity to existing treatment programs generally displayed by cases in which there is a greater degree of differentiation. It may be pointed out, however, that these forms are very sensitive to cortisone, whether alone or in combinations; with the doses now employed, this drug is also active against lymphoblasts outside the cycle.

Lastly, it is not yet known if and to what extent immunological treatment is able to prevent the recruitment of resting blasts by imprisoning them in this stage. A mechanism of this kind, however, would serve to explain the greater effectiveness of immunotherapy in the more differentiated forms of the disease, since, as our present inquiry has shown, it is here that the number of quiescent blasts is considerably higher than in other forms.

References

1. Gavosto, F.: Kinetics of human acute leukaemia — The kinetics of cellular proliferation, p. 291. Paris: M. Tubiana, Ed. I.N.S.E.R.M. (1971).
2. Gavosto, F.: The proliferative kinetics of the acute leukemias in relation to their treatment. Europ. J. clin. biol. Res. **10**, 1042 (1970).
3. Gavosto, F., Pileri, A., Bachi, C., Pegoraro, L.: Proliferation and maturation defect in acute leukaemia cells. Nature (Lond.) **203**, 92 (1964).
4. Gavosto, F., Pileri, A., Gabutti, V., Masera, P.: Non selfmaintaining kinetics of proliferating blasts in human acute leukaemia. Nature (Lond.) **216**, 188 (1967 a).
5. Gavosto, F., Pileri, A., Gabutti, V., Masera, P.: Cell population kinetics in human acute leukaemia. Europ. J. Cancer **3**, 301 (1967 b).

Cytokinetic Studies and Treatment Response in Adult Acute Leukemia

E. Frei, III and Jacqueline S. Hart

Texas Medical Center, Anderson Hospital, Houston, TX/USA

Introduction

There is increasing emphasis on cytokinetic studies as a basis for constructing treatment programs for cancer. In the present study various pretreatment cytokinetic factors were analyzed with respect to their correlation with response to treatment and prognosis.

Methods

Sixty-eight adults with acute leukemia admitted consecutively to the University of Texas, M. D. Anderson Hospital and Tumor Institute, were studied. The distribution of the patients by morphologic type of leukemia, prior treatment, and various cytokinetic and response characteristics is presented in Table 1.

Table 1. Summary of pretherapy variables, response, and survival

Variables	AML		ALL		
	No Prior Rx	Prior Rx	No Prior Rx	Prior Rx	Total patients
Labeling index %	11	10	14	16	12
% absolute marrow infiltrate	55	53	91	81	61
Absolute blasts in blood (×10³)	2.5	1.5	13.5	7.0	2.4
Age (years)	49	42	31	18	41
Complete remission No. (%) [a]	14 (41%)	7 (50%)	7 (58%)	0 (0%)	28 (41%)
Duration (months)	9	5	6	—	7
Survival — months from diagnosis	4.5	20.5	9.5	23.5	9
1st cytokinetic study	4	5.5	9.5	5.5	6
Total no. patients [a]	34	14	12	8	68

[a] Values expressed are medians except for those marked.

The percentage of leukemic cells (blast cells and promyclocytes in AML) was determined from the marrow smear. The cellularity of the marrow was estimated by visual scanning and Chalkly counts of the marrow section (clot or biopsy). The percentage of absolute marrow infiltrate was defined as the product of the percentage of leukemic cells determined from the smear differential and the % cellularity of the marrow particle as determined by section [1].

The labeling index (LI %) was determined as follows: a marrow aspirate was obtained and a single cell suspension was prepared. It was incubated in Eagles minimal essential medium at a concentration of 1×10^6 cells for one hour following the addition of five microcurie of tritiated thymidine. After one hour a cell pellet was obtained and autoradiographs were prepared (for details, see ref. 2).

Results

A summary of the pretreatment variables and response is presented in Table 1. The % absolute marrow infiltrate was significantly higher in patients with ALL than for patients with AML ($P = 0.01$). The pretreatment LI % was somewhat, though not significantly, higher in ALL patients. The relationship between pretreatment leukemic cell LI and other variables for patients with AML is presented in Fig. 1. There was a significant and positive correlation between the LI % and the % absolute marrow infiltrate. There was a significant negative correlation between age and % absolute

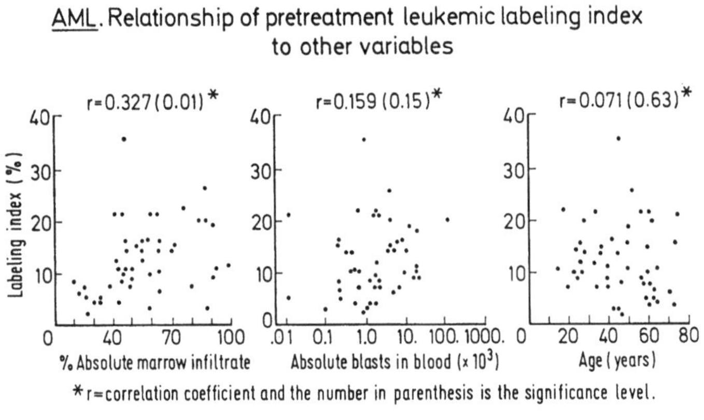

Fig. 1

marrow infiltrate in AML ($p = 0.05$). A similar relationship held for ALL but could not be quantified because the number of patients was smaller. Since age is a major factor influencing prognosis in AML, partial correlation coefficients were performed keeping age constant. It was found that the positive correlation between LI % and % absolute marrow infiltrate was independent of age for both AML and ALL.

The relationship of the pretreatment LI %, the % absolute marrow infiltrate and age to response for patients with AML is presented in Table 2. There was a significant increase in the complete remission rate with an increasing LI % and a significant decrease in the complete remission rate with increasing age. Although not statistically

Table 2. AML — Relationship of pretherapy variables to response

Response	Labelling index %			% Absolute marrow infiltrate			Age (years)		
	≦ 8	9—15	≧ 16	< 50	50—75	> 75	≦ 30	31—50	≧ 50
	No. pts. (%)	No. pts. (%)	No. pts. (%)	No. pts. (%)	No. pts. (%)	No. pts. (%)	No. pts. (%)	No. pts. (%)	No. pts. (%)
CR [a]	3 (18)	9 (53)	9 (64)	7 (30)	10 (67)	4 (40)	7 (64)	9 (56)	5 (24)
NR	14 (82)	8 (47)	5 (36)	16 (70)	5 (33)	6 (60)	4 (36)	7 (44)	16 (76)
Total no. patients	17	17	14	23	15	10	11	16	21
Chi square	$p < 0.01$			$p = 0.13$			$p < 0.05$		

[a] CR = Complete remission
NR = No response or partial remission

Table 3. AML — Relationship of pretherapy variables to response for separate age groups

Response	< 50 years				≧ 50 years			
	Labelling index %		% Absolute marrow infiltrate		Labelling index %		% Absolute marrow infiltrate	
	≦ 8 Pts. (%)	> 8 Pts. (%)	< 50 Pts. (%)	≧ 50 Pts. (%)	≦ 8 Pts. (%)	> 8 Pts. (%)	< 50 Pts. (%)	≧ 50 Pts. (%)
CR [a]	3 (33)	13 (72)	7 (64)	9 (56)	0 (0)	5 (38)	0 (0)	5 (56)
NR	6 (67)	5 (28)	4 (36)	7 (44)	8 (100)	8 (62)	12 (100)	4 (44)
Total no. patients	9	18	11	16	8	13	12	9
Fisher's exact test	p = 0.13		p = 0.98		p = 0.14		p = 0.02	

[a] CR = Complete remission
NR = No response or partial remission

significant there was a positive relationship between the % absolute marrow infiltrate with complete remission. The same general trends obtained for ALL.

Since age is known to affect response to treatment, an effort was made to determine whether the LI % and the % absolute marrow infiltrate correlated with response to treatment independent of age (Table 3). Patients under the age of 50 with a high LI % (greater than 8) had a complete remission rate of 72% compared to 33% for those with a low LI %. For patients over the age of 50, the complete remission rate was 38% for those with a high LI % and 0 for those with a low LI %. Thus, though the complete remission rate was lower in patients over the age of 50 the positive correlation between response and LI % was independent of age. Again, the same trend obtained for patients with ALL but the numbers were too small for quantitative comparison.

The relationship of pretreatment cytokinetics to the duration of complete remission of patients with AML is presented in Table 4. There was a negative correlation between the duration of complete remission and the labelling index. Thus, for patients with low labelling indices (less than 8) the medium duration of remission was 17 months: for intermediate labelling indices (9 to 15%) 12.5 months; and for high labelling indices (greater than 16) five months.

Table 4. AML — Relationship of pretherapy variables to median duration of complete remission

	Labelling index %			% Absolute marrow infiltrate			Age (years)		
Duration of complete remission	$\leqq 8$	9—15	$\geqq 16$	< 50	50—75	> 75	$\leqq 30$	31—50	$\geqq 50$
Median in months	17	12.5	5.0	17	6	4	6	18	7.5
Total no. patients	3	9	9	7	10	4	7	9	5

Discussion

For both morphological types of acute leukemia, and particularly AML, there was a significant positive correlation between the LI % and the % absolute marrow infiltrate. It has been observed that when patients are studied early in relapse, when the degree of leukemic cell infiltration of the marrow is low, the LI % is high and tends to decrease as the marrow infiltrate increases [3—6]. This is consistent with experimental *in vivo* and *in vitro* studies where both the growth fraction and cell loss increased with increasing tumor size and tumor cell concentration [7—9]. Our studies on the other hand were conducted in patients who presumably were on the flat or plateau portion of the growth curve. It seems reasonable that leukemias with a high proliferative "thrust", that is, were a greater proportion of the cells are in DNA synthesis (LI %), would be associated with a greater degree of bone marrow displacement by the leukemic cells. In fact, if one examines Fig. 1, it appears that the LI %

increases as the % absolute marrow infiltrate increased from 20 to 50%, after which there is no further increase in the LI %.

There was a significant negative correlation between age and % absolute marrow infiltrative. Also, there was a negative correlation between age and the LI %. This is consistent with the observation that AML in elderly patients seems to be less "aggressive" and also less responsive to chemotherapy [10—11]. Since age has been established as a significant factor in prognosis, the relationship between the cytokinetic variables independent of age was examined. It was found that the LI % and the % absolute marrow infiltrate were positively correlated, independent of age ($P = 0.05$). There is evidence in some neoplastic diseases that the proliferative capacity decreases with age [12—13]. In human and experimental systems, it has been demonstrated that the normal bone marrow reserve decreases with age [14]. Our observations that the % absolute marrow infiltrate tends to be lower in the elderly is consistent with the above. However, in this analysis the proliferative "thrust" (LI %) of the disease was found to be independent of age, as indicated in Table 3, where 18 of 27 patients under the age of 50 had a LI % of greater than 8, and 13 of 21 patients over the age of 50 had a LI % of greater than 8.

There was a positive correlation between the LI % and the response to treatment in terms of the complete remission rate, which was independent of age. Since most chemotherapeutic agents affect primarily proliferating cells, it is not surprising that there is a positive correlation between the initial response and the proportion of cells undergoing DNA synthesis. The high LI % is a function primarily of a high Ts/Tc ratio (total time in DNA synthesis divided by intermitotic time) and a high growth fraction. Both would favor responsiveness to chemotherapy.

Of great interest is the observation that, though there was a positive correlation between complete remission rate and the LI %, there was a negative correlation between the duration of complete remission and the LI %. This is consistent with the fact that the faster the cell turnover the greater the opportunity for the selection of resistant cells, and the more rapid the increase in the number of cells when chemotherapy is no longer effective. In general, the same cytokinetic factors which lead initially to an increase in the magnitude of cell destruction (remission induction) increase the rate at which relapse occurs (remission maintenance).

These observations have implications for the tactics of remission maintenance chemotherapy. Thus, for patients with high LI % and other evidence of rapid cell turnover, the intervals between treatment should be as short as possible during early remission. The general practice has been to progressively increase the interval between courses of treatment to one month for patients in remission. While this may be appropriate for patients with low proliferative thrust, it is inadequate for patients with high LI % and different tactics are indicated.

References

1. HART, J. S., DONNER, R. S., GEHAN, E., FREIREICH, E. J.: Cellularity — A method for evaluation of marrow response to chemotherapy in adult acute leukemia (AAL). Proc. Amer. Ass. Cancer Res. 11, 34 (1970).
2. HART, J. S., GEORGE, S. L., NICKERSON, R. C., FREI, E. III.: Cytokinetic studies and clinical correlations in adult acute leukemia. Blood. (In press.)
3. KILLMAN, S. A.: The kinetics of leukemic blast cells in man. Ser. Haemat. 1, 38 (1968).

4. MAUER, A. M., SAUNDERS, E. F., LAMPKIN, B. C.: The nature and causes of the variability of proliferative activity in marrow cell populations in acute leukemia: The Proliferation and Spread of Neoplastic Cells, M. D. Anderson Hospital Symposium, pp. 359—368. Baltimore: William and Wilkins Co. 1968.
5. CLARKSON, B. D., FRIED, J.: Changing concepts of treatment in acute leukemia. Med. Clin. N. Amer. **55**, 561—597 (1971).
6. CLARKSON, B., TODO, A., OGAWA, M., GEE, T., FRIED, J.: Consideration of the cell cycle in chemotherapy of acute leukemia: Recent Results of Cancer Research. New York: Springer 1971.
7. SKIPPER, H. E.: Prediction of response to cancer therapy. Nat. Cancer Inst. Monogr. **33**, pp. 2—14, 1970.
8. TODO, A., STRIFE, A., FRIED, J. CLARKSON, B.: Proliferative kinetics of human hematopoietic cells during different growth phases *in vitro*. Cancer Res. **31**, 1330—1340 (1971).
9. FRIED, J. A.: A mathematical model to aid in the interpretation of radioactive tracer data from proliferating cell populations. Math. Biosciences **8**, 379—396 (1970).
10. FREIREICH, E. J., BODEY, G. P., HARRIS, J. E., HART, J. S.: Therapy for acute granulocytic leukemia. Cancer Res. **27**, 2573—2577 (1967).
11. GEE, T. S., YU, K. P., CLARKSON, B. D.: Treatment of adult acute leukemia with arabinosyl cytosine and thioguanine. Cancer (Philad.) **23**, 1019 (1969).
12. PAPADRIANOS, E., COOLEY, E., HOAGENSON, C. D.: Mammary carcinoma in old age. Ann. Surg. **161**, 189—194 (1965).
13. ALEXANIAN, R.: Multiple Myeloma: A nine-year experience with melphalan therapy at the M. D. Anderson Hospital. Leukemia-lymphoma — The 14th annual clinical conference on Cancer, 1969, at the University of Texas, M. D. Anderson Hospital, pp. 305—316, Yearbook Publishers, 1969.
14. HARTSOCK, R. J., SMITH, E. B., PETTY, C. S.: Normal variations with aging of the amount of hematopoietic tissue in bone marrow from the anterior iliac crest. Amer. J. clin. Path. **43**, 326—331 (1965).

Contribution of Cultures in Agar to the Classification of Acute Leukemias: Preliminary Results *

P. Pouillart

Institut de Cancérologie et d' Immunogénétique **, Hôpital Paul-Brousse ***, Villejuif/France

In a previous work with Mathé *et al.* [1], we subdivided acute lymphoid leukemia (ALL) and acute myeloid leukemia (AML) into subtypes, the identification of which is based on an analysis of the morphological features of the marrow cell elements obtained prior to treatment and stained with May Grunwald Giemsa (MGG).

Although the differences between the most highly differentiated cell types of AML and ALL are clearcut, they are much less distinct between the elements of the less differentiated forms, namely the so-called "promyeloblastic" (PMbAL) and "prolymphoblastic" (PLbAL) subvarieties. These two types have probably been confused for a long time because of their imprecise classification; yet their chemical sensitivity to the drugs used for remission induction or maintenance, and their prognosis are different.

In vitro methods of growing colonies by bone marrow culture in semi-solid media have been much used for the study of hemopoietic stem cells [2, 3, 4]. Such systems have already demonstrated the possibility of obtaining colonies from leukemic blast cells of myeloid origin taken from a patient in the clinically evident phase of the disease before any treatment has been initiated [4, 5, 6, 7]. Colony growth and the differentiation of blast cells can be accomplished only when the cultures are stimulated in vitro, either by a feeder layer of normal circulating granulocytes [6] or by a conditioned medium obtained from a culture of human spleen cells or, finally, in the presence of semi-purified urinary factors [3].

Material and Methods

The method we have used is that of Robinson [6] (see Fig. 1).

The sublayer is prepared immediately prior to use. In a semi-solid medium of 0.5% agar, 2×10^6 circulating leucocytes of a normal donor are immobilized at a temperature of 38° C; 2 ml of this preparation is allowed to solidify in a 35 mm diameter Petri dish. The growth layer consists of a semi-solid medium of 0.3% agar in

* We gratefully acknowledge that this work was made possible through a grant given by the Faculty of Medicine, Paris Sud.

** INSERM et Association Claude-Bernard

*** 14—16, avenue Paul-Vaillant Couturier

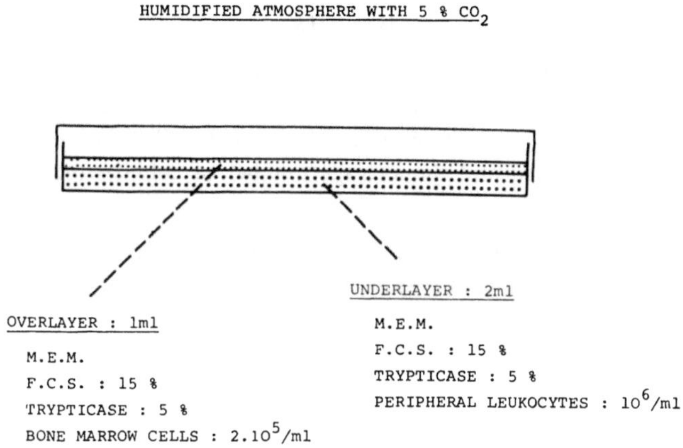

Fig. 1. Scheme representing the technique used for agar culture

which are immobilized 2×10^5 bone marrow cells per ml, washed twice in culture medium. One ml of this preparation is placed on the growth layer. The medium used for the preparation of the sublayer and the growth layer is culture medium enriched with 5% trypticase and 15% fetal calf serum. The Petri dish is then placed in an incubator at 37° C in a humidified atmosphere containing 5% CO_2. The reading is made on the twentieth day of incubation. The dishes were scored for "clusters" or "agglomerates" of fewer than 50 cells and "colonies" of more than 50 cells (Fig. 2).

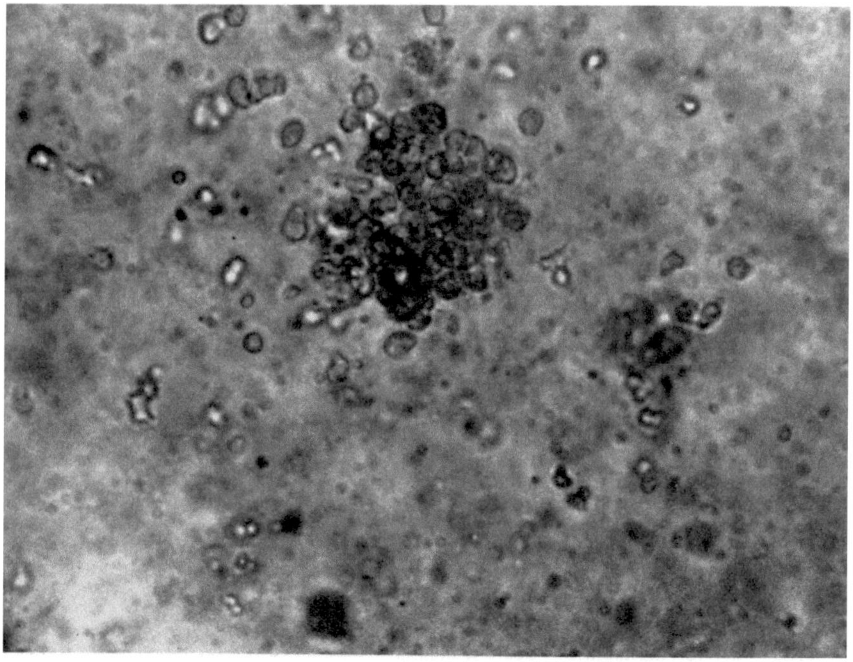

Fig. 2. Morphological aspect of colonies in agar

Results

The number of colonies obtained for each of the classical varieties of acute leukemia is given in Table 1. These results represent an average of the cases studied, each point being determined by averaging at least five incubated dishes. Five normal marrow specimens were studied and the average number of colonies established for each

Table 1. Average number of colonies and clusters obtained by agar culture according to the cytological type of bone marrow cultured

1. *Normal bone marrow*	Colonies	64
	Clusters	140
2. *Acute myeloid leukemia*	Colonies	143
	Clusters	120
"promyeloblastic"	Colonies	200
	Clusters	160
3. *Acute lymphoid leukemia*	Colonies	4
	Clusters	47
"prolymphoblastic"	Colonies	5
	Clusters	41

Table 2. Number of colonies and clusters according to the cytological type of acute leukemia bone marrow cultured

		Number of colonies	Number of clusters
Normal bone marrow		46	157
		81	142
		65	135
		63	127
		69	141
A. L. L.	PLbAL	0	32
	PLbAL	11	117
	PLbAL	10	16
	PLbAL	0	—
	MLbAL *	0	—
	MLbAL	13	—
	MLbAL	1	16
	PLcAL *	15	16
	ALL (in partial remission)	60	—
A. M. L.	PMbAL	207	—
	PMbAL	192	160
	AML	100	—
	AML	76	81

* MLbAL="macrolymphoblastic" acute leukemia
* PLcAL="prolymphocytic" acute leukemia

200,000 cells cultured was 64. For colonies obtained from ALL bone marrow the average was 4, while it was 143 for the AML cultures.

The colonies observed are often smaller in size than colonies obtained under the same conditions with normal human bone marrow. Their morphological evolution is identical. Beside typical colonies, clusters or groups with 8—50 cells have been counted. Colonies are more frequent in the cultures of bone marrow from AML patients than in ALL cultures. For ALL the number of colonies is below normal for each cytological variety and remains, in all cases, less than 15, while with AML cells, the number of colonies is higher than the number obtained from normal bone marrow. Furthermore, there is a significant difference between the results obtained with the most immature or "promyeloblastic" varieties (an average of 200 colonies) and the most highly differentiated or "promyelocytic" varieties, where the average number of colonies obtained is 90 (Table 2).

Discussion

The number of patients studied is too small to allow reliable conclusions, especially on the nature of the cells which give rise to the colonies and clusters. Our work continues and will be complemented by the use of chromosomal markers when these are available.

Our results could, however, be useful for recognizing ALL and AML, which are difficult to distinguish by means of light microscopy. We must, however, underline that the number of AML patients is so small that we cannot assume that the larger number of colonies found in this preliminary work is constant and could be helpful in characterizing this disease. The constancy of the smaller number of colonies produced by ALL bone marrow is more probable, owing to the greater number of ALL patients studied.

References

1. Mathé, G., Pouillart, P., Sterescu, M., Amiel, J. L., Schwarzenberg, L., Schneider, M., Hayat, M., De Vassal, F., Jasmin, C., Lafleur, M.: Subdivision of classical varieties of acute leukemia. Correlation with prognosis and cure expectancy. Europ. J. clin. biol. Res. **16**, 554 (1971).
2. Pluznik, D. H., Sachs, L.: The cloning in normal mast cells in tissue culture. J. cell. comp. Physiol. **72**, 251 (1965).
3. Broodley, T. R., Metcalf, D.: The growth of mouse bone marrow cells in vitro. Aust. J. exp. Biol. med. Sci. **44**, 287 (1966).
4. Ichikawa, Y.: Differentiation of a cell line of myeloid leukemia. J. cell. comp. Physiol. **74**, 223 (1969).
5. Metcalf, D., Moore, M. A. S.: Factors modifying stem cell proliferation of myelomonocytic leukemic cells in vitro and in vivo. J. nat. Cancer Inst. **44**, 801 (1970).
6. Kurnick, J. E., Robinson, W. A.: Colony growth of human peripheral white blood cells in vitro. Blood **37**, 136 (1971).
7. Iscove, N. N., Senn, J. S., Till, J. E., McCulloch, E. A.: Colony formation by normal and leukemic human marrow cells in culture. Effect of conditioned medium from human leucocytes. Blood **37**, 1 (1971).

The Heterogeneity of Cell Culture Findings in Patients with Acute Myeloblastic Leukemia*

D. H. Cowan, H. A. Messner, J. S. Senn, and E. A. McCulloch

Department of Medicine, Princess Margaret Hospital and the Ontario Cancer Institute and Sunnybrook Hospital and the University of Toronto, Toronto/Canada

The availability of a colony-forming culture assay that detects early progenitors of granulopoiesis (colony forming units in culture; CFU-C) in human bone marrow cells [1, 2, 4, 5, 8, 9, 10] makes it possible to study cellular events in leukemia. Although the CFU-C culture method does not assay directly for the pluripotent myeloid stem cell, there is ample evidence that cells giving rise to colonies in culture are progeny of the pluripotent stem cell and may provide information about early cellular events (for review, see [7]). Marrow suspensions from adult patients with untreated acute myeloblastic leukemia were examined. The results indicate that there are at least several subtypes; this supports the view that the disease we call acute myeloblastic leukemia (AML) is mechanistically heterogeneous.

Materials and Methods

Patients

Material was obtained from patients of the acute leukemia service of the Princess Margaret Hospital and the haematology service of Sunnybrook Hospital. Data are presented only for patients who had received no previous antileukemic therapy. Subsequent treatment consisted of intensive four-day courses of cyclophosphamide, arabinosyl cytosine and vincristine (CAV protocol) [3] repeated each two to three weeks, unless otherwise specified. Patients whose marrow cells showed some differentiation to monocytes (acute myelomonocytic leukemia; AMMOL) were included in the broad category of AML. Serum and urine muramidase levels were determined on 22 of the patients [1].

Cell Culture

The culture method was a modification of the method of Iscove *et al.* [6]. Bone marrow suspensions were centrifuged for ten minutes at 150 g and the buffy coat

---

* Supported by research grants from the Ontario Cancer Treatment and Research Foundation and Medical Research Council of Canada

1 Muramidase determinations were performed by Dr. Waldemar Pruzanski of the Wellesley Hospital, by the lysoplate method of Osserman and Lawlor.

removed. After two washes in tissue culture medium [11] appropriate numbers of nucleated cells were plated in methyl cellulose with or without 20% "conditioned medium" (colony stimulating activity; CSA) prepared from normal peripheral blood leukocytes [5]. The cultures also contained alpha medium [11] and 20% fetal calf serum. Cultures were incubated at 37° C in a moist atmosphere containing 7.5% CO_2. The cultures may be assessed on the basis of number of colonies (20 cells or greater), colony size, colony morphology and variations dependent on presence or absence of CSA. The results reported in this paper have been accumulated over a period of 2½ years. During this time, the detailed assessment of the colonies has been extended; consequently all parameters are not available for every patient.

Results

Data are available for 25 patients with untreated AML. The results are shown in the Table. The cells from 21 of the patients (Group A) behaved in a similar manner. Little or no growth occurred without CSA. The addition of 20% CSA resulted in a modest increase in the number of small colonies as previously reported [3], but in no cases did the number of colonies reach our normal values of 80—120/10^5 nucleated cells plated. The majority of these colonies could be identified as granulocytic. Fig. 1 shows the culture results, with CSA, for these 21 patients as a function of the percentage of blast cells in the same aspirate. It should be noted that colony-forming efficiency bore no relationship to the percentage of blast cells in the marrow, or to the response to subsequent treatment with CAV. Muramidase levels were available on serum and/or urine of 18 patients and in 9 cases the values were elevated. There was no difference in the colony-forming efficiency of the cells cultured with CSA from those patients with elevated and normal muramidase levels.

There were two patients in Group B. The colony-forming efficiency of the marrow cells from both fell within, or close to, our normal range, and the addition of 20% CSA did not have a great effect. The colonies from one patient (B-2) were almost all macrophage colonies. Unfortunately, the analysis of colony type was not carried out on the other patient (B-1). Patient B-1 responded to CAV in an incomplete manner. She never achieved complete remission, although there was marked improve-

Table. Colony-forming efficiency of marrow cells from 25 patients with untreated AML

No.	Patients	CFU/10^5 Nucleated Cells		Colony Morphology
		Without CSA	With CSA	
A.	21	Range 0—27 Median 2	Range 0—65 Median 10	Mainly granulocytic
B.	B-1	96	96	Not done
	B-2	74	122	All macrophage
C.	C-1	> 1,000	> 1,000	80% granulocytic
	C-2	> 1,000	> 1,000	

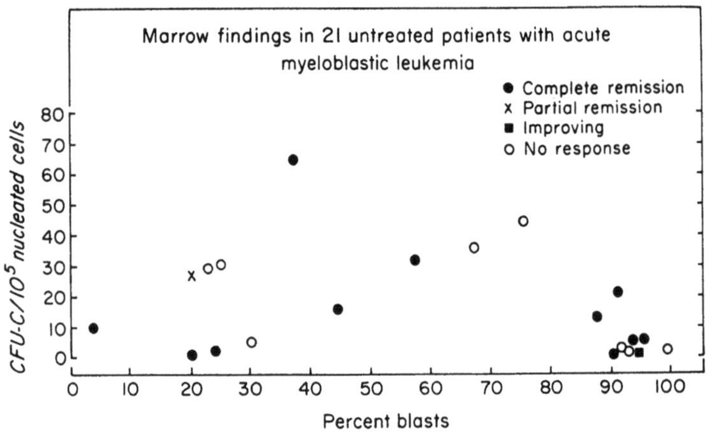

Fig. 1. Marrow findings in 21 untreated patients (Group A) with untreated AML. Patients who subsequently achieved remission, patients progressing toward remission, and patients unresponsive to CAV treatment are shown

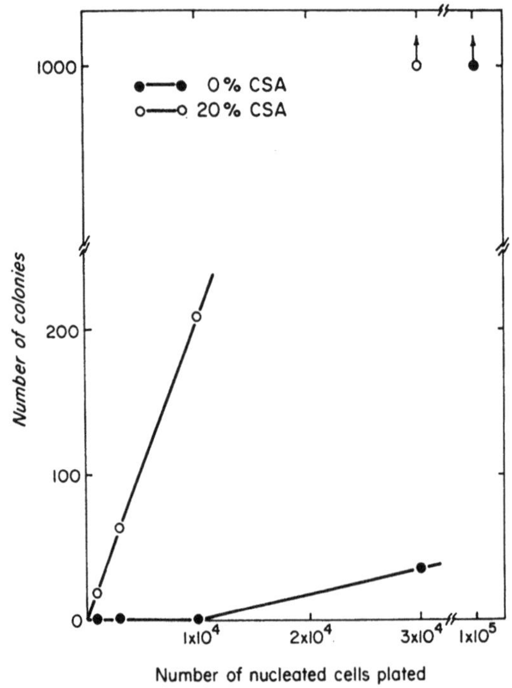

Fig. 2. Colony-forming efficiency of marrow cells from patient C-1, plated at different cell numbers (10^3—10^5) with and without CSA. Note break in scale for cell numbers greater than 3×10^4

ment in her peripheral blood counts and she survived 13 months after diagnosis. Patient B-2 failed to respond to six courses of CAV and died 15 weeks after diagnosis. Muramidase levels were normal in both patients.

The cells from two patients (Group C) behaved in an unusual fashion. When 10^5 bone marrow cells were plated, growth was confluent both with and without 20% CSA. However, at lower cell concentrations ($10^3-3\times10^4$), there was a marked difference in growth with and without CSA. Fig. 2 shows this effect for one of the patients (C-1). The colonies in both cases were granulocytic. Patient C-1 is a 78-year-old man who presented with anaemia, granulocytopenia, a small number of blast cells in the peripheral blood, and a bone marrow aspirate containing 43% myeloblasts. Muramidase levels were normal. He has not received any antileukemic therapy and continues to be managed, nine months after diagnosis, with intermittent blood transfusions. Patient C-2 was a 63-year-old man with more than 50,000 blast cells per mm^3 in the peripheral blood and gross infiltration of the bone marrow with blast cells. The muramidase level was elevated. He received two courses of CAV without response, and died of a myocardial infarct 5 weeks after diagnosis.

Discussion

We do not suggest that the grouping of patients provided in this paper should form a basis of classification of AML. Rather, the culture results provide an indication that such a classification may become possible when more patients have been studied and the significance of changes in CFU-C are understood in relationship to their postulated pluripotent progenitors. From this point of view, the present data represent the "tip of the iceberg". Further developments may yield a classification of acute myeloblastic leukemia with a mechanistic basis similar to that now available for the megaloblastic states.

References

1. Brown, D. H., (III), Carbone, P. P.: *In vitro* growth of normal and leukemic bone marrow. J. nat. Cancer Inst. **46**, 989 (1971).
2. Chervenick, P. A., Boggs, E. R.: Bone marrow colonies: Stimulation *in vitro* by supernatant from incubated human blood cells. Science **169**, 692 (1971).
3. Cowan, D. H., Clarysse, A., Abu-Zahra, H., Senn, J. S., McCulloch, E. A.: The effect of remission induction in acute myeloblastic leukemia on efficiency of colony formation in culture. Ser. Haemat. V. **2**, 105 (1972).
4. Greenberg, P. C., Nichols, W. C., Schrier, S. L.: Granulopoiesis in acute myeloid leukemia and pre-leukemia. New. Engl. J. Med. **284**, 1225 (1971).
5. Iscove, N. N., Senn, J. S., Till, J. S., McCulloch, E. A.: Colony formation by normal and leukemic human marrow cells in culture: Effect of conditioned medium from leukocytes. Blood **37**, 1 (1971).
6. Iscove, N. N., Messner, H., Till, J. E., McCulloch, E. A.: Human marrow cells forming colonies in culture: Analysis by velocity sedimentation and suspension culture. Ser. Haemat. V. **2**, 37 (1972).
7. McCulloch, E. A., Till, J. E.: Leukemia considered as defective differentiation: Complementary *in vivo* and culture methods applied to the clinical problem. The Nature of Leukemia, p. 119. Ed.: P. C. Vincent. Sydney, Australia: V. C. N. Blight, Government Printer.

8. MOORE, M. A. S., WILLIAMS, N., METCALFE, D.: Characterization of *in vitro* colony-forming cells in acute and chronic myeloid leukemia. The Nature of Leukemia, p. 135. Ed.: P. C. VINCENT. Sydney, Australia: V. C. N. Blight, Government Printer.
9. PIKE, B. L., ROBINSON, W. A.: Human bone marrow colony growth in agar-gel. J. cell. comp. Physiol. **76**, 77 (1970).
10. SENN, J. S., MCCULLOCH, E. A., TILL, J. E.: Comparison of colony-forming ability of normal and leukemic human marrow in cell culture. Lancet **1967 II**, 597.
11. STANNERS, C. P., ELICEIRI, G. L., GREEN, H.: Synthesis of ribosomal RNA in mouse-hamster hybrids. Nature (Lond.) (New Biol.) **250**, 52 (1971).

Biochemical Techniques for Classification of Leukemic Cell Types*

T. C. Hall, D. Kessel, A. Nahas, and B. Hacker

American Cancer Society Research Professor RP-42, Division of Oncology, University of Rochester Medical Center, Rochester, NY/USA

Introduction

We are quite accustomed to having two virtually identical leukemic blast cells respond entirely differently to a chemotherapeutic drug or drug combination. In fact, it is easier to find meaningful dissimilarity in the drug response of leukemic blasts than to distinguish meaningful morphologic similarity. We know that for a drug to destroy a leukemic blast several things are required:

1. The drug must be transported into the cell;
2. in many instances it must be anabolized by the cell into an active form;
3. an adequate biochemical target must be present in the cell;
4. no alternative pathways to the blocked one can be present, otherwise the drug-inhibited pathway will not create a lethal defect.

We have looked at normal granulocytes and lymphocytes, and the abnormal cells of acute and chronic leukemias, with respect to ability to transport drugs, their complement of drug-metabolizing enzymes, and the rates at which they synthesize nucleic acids. Although these studies are still incomplete, they provide evidence that major cell types can be distinguished from each other by biochemical techniques. In addition, these studies suggest that it may be possible to distinguish potentially drug-sensitive cells from resistant cells.

Fig. 1 shows the differences between cell types in respect to methotrexate (MTX) transport. There are marked differences between normal small lymphocytes and granulocytes. The small lymphocytes of CLL behave like normal small lymphocytes, and some granulocytes of acute and chronic myelogeneous leukemia resemble normal granulocytes. Some blast cells, whether lymphatic or myelogenous, take up as much methotrexate as normal cells; those which take up a lot of MTX can be as sensitive to the drug as normal granulocyte precursors, while those blasts that take up as little MTX as a small lymphocyte are equally unaffected by it [1].

6-Mercaptopurine (6MP), like the other purine and pyrimidine analogs, requires phosphorylation to an active compound in order to become effective. Fig. 2 shows that, again, small lymphocytes are relatively inactive, and normal granulocytes are

* Supported in part by NCI Grant Ca 11198.

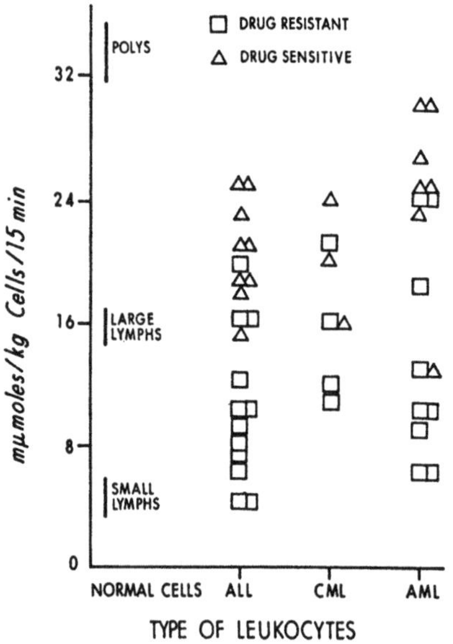

Fig. 1. Methotrexate transport by different white cells and leukemia cell types

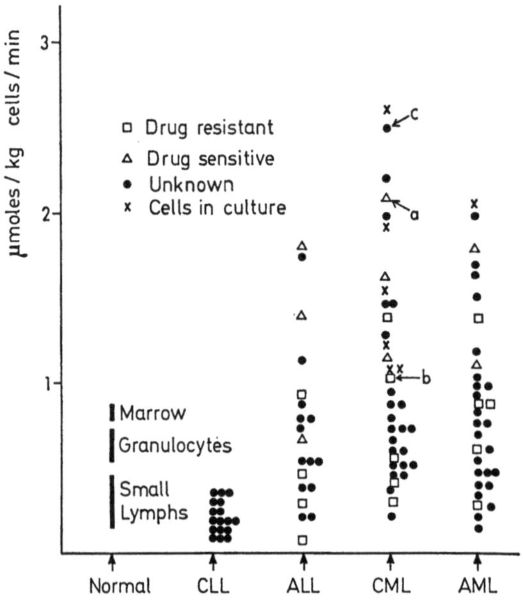

Fig. 2 a—c. Phosphorylation by different leukemia cell types of 6 MP. a Patient untreated, b Same patient after treatment with 6-MP, response, and development of drug resistance, c Same patient one year later

moderately active. As before, the cells of the chronic leukemias resemble their normal precursors in a striking manner. Acute leukemic blast cells are more variable, but the highly drug-sensitive cells are readily distinguishable from those resistant to the drug [2].

A similar situation exists for cytarabine (CA), but there are marked differences (Fig. 3). CA is extensively phosphorylated by small lymphocytes, and in this respect is different from all other antimetabolites [3]. This high level of phosphorylation permits a CLL cell or normal lymphocyte to be readily distinguished. CA can be deaminated, although the leukemic cellular concentration of deaminase is unrelated

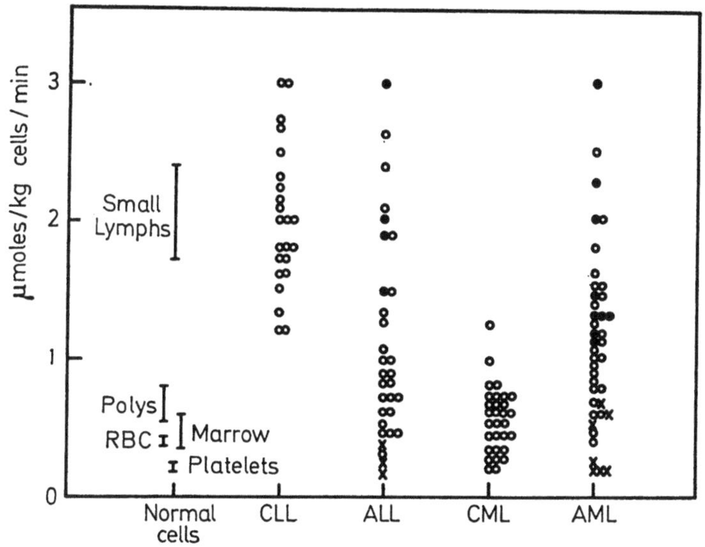

Fig. 3. Phosphorylation, by different leukemia and normal cell types, of cytarabine

to its drug sensitivity [4]. There are, however, marked differences in the amount of deaminase present in different cell types, as can be seen from Fig. 4: granulocytes generally have much more enzyme than lymphocytes while blast cells have relatively little [5].

Workers using thymidine labeling techniques have reported finding very little DNA synthesis in the circulating leukocytes in the serum. This is consistent with the concept that a degree of irreversible maturation must precede release from the marrow. Blast cells, on the other hand, would be expected to show a considerable amount of DNA synthesis. We were surprised to find a considerable amount of DNA synthesis in chronic myelogenous leukemias too, even when few or no frank blasts were circulating [6].

We have constructed a number of cell profiles. Fig. 5 shows a normal population of mixed white cells, about 75% of which are granulocytes. This profile was compiled from data on specific patients; it is included as a faint dotted line on the subsequent profiles. If this profile is compared with that for small lymphocytes from CLL patients (Fig. 6), it will be seen to resemble the profile of small lymphocytes from

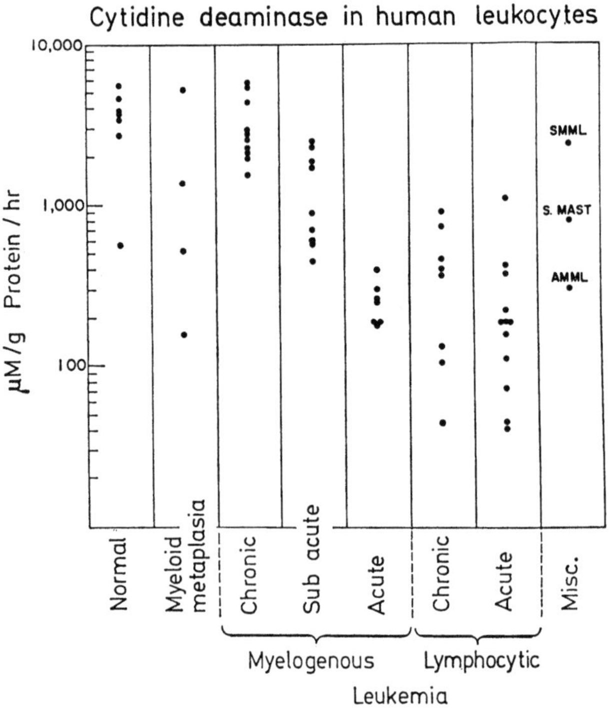

Fig. 4

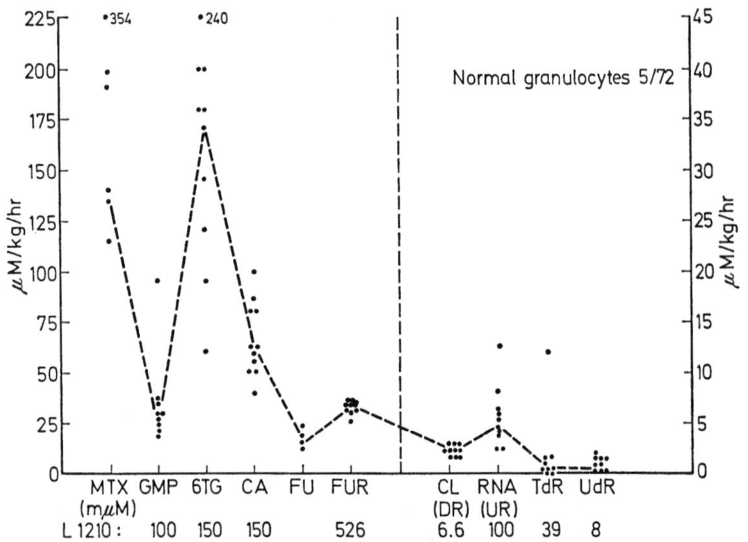

Fig. 5. Profile of normal leukocyte population showing drug uptakes and nucleic acid synthesis rates

normal blood. However, the lack of methotrexate transport and the large amount of cytarabine phosphorylation stand in marked contrast to the first cell type. As can be seen from Table, the ability to phosphorylate cytarabine is more developed in human lymphocytes than in those of other species, and might perhaps form the basis for an as yet unexploited immunosuppressive function of cytarabine. The differences in the cytarabine phosphorylation capacity of lymphocytes of different origin suggests a biochemical classification of cells by species and organ of origin. Another important biochemical discriminant, which is not shown here, is deoxycytidine deaminase; the level of this enzyme is very high in granulocytes and quite low in small lymphocytes.

The cells of CML patients (Fig. 7) should be and are similar to normal granulocytes in their MTX and cycloleucine transport functions. However, in many cells both RNA and DNA synthesis are markedly higher than in normal granulocytes. Some of the other DNA-synthesizing enzymes, such as thymidine kinase, responsible for activation of the antileukemic analogs are also elevated in CML.

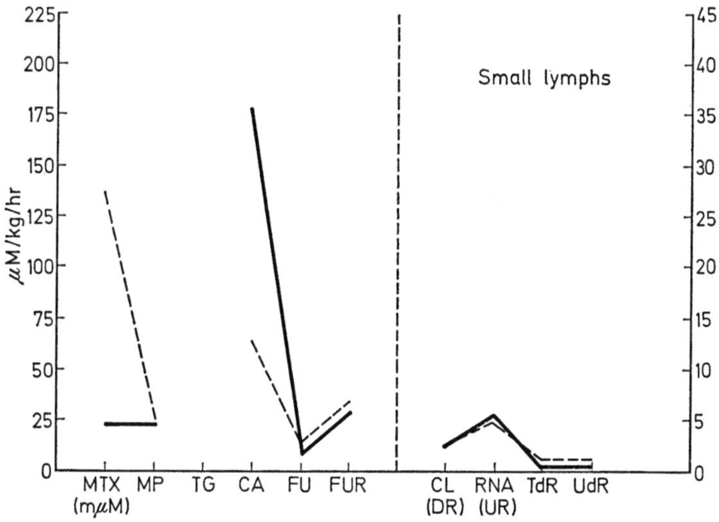

Fig. 6. Profile of small lymphocytes from CLL patients, (light line represents normal mixed peripheral leukocytes)

Table. Lymphocytes by cytarabine phosphorylation in different species

	Expressed as % of human blood lymphocytes			
Species	Thymus	Spleen	Lymph node	Blood
Mouse	68	11	11	26
Rat	65	17	16	18
Dog	109	6	6	5
Rabbit	176	11	32	32
Rhesus monkey	100	48	39	22

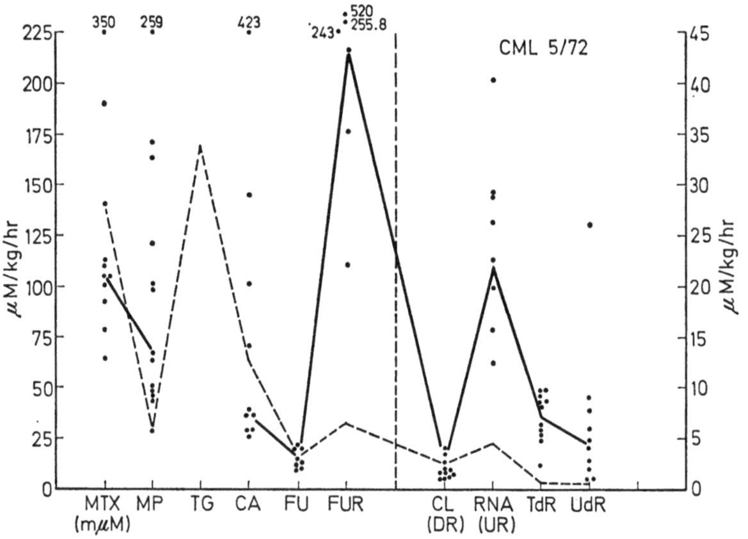

Fig. 7. Profile of granulocytes from CML patients

Cells from AML patients, as shown on the next Fig. 8, differ from their normal and chronic leukemia homologues in their DNA-synthesizing activity. Interestingly, they also tend to make more RNA.

Fig. 9 is a semidiagrammatic composite of the data presented in Figs. 5—8. In the case of the acute leukemic cells, those which phosphorylate a drug well are commonly found to have extensive drug-induced inhibitions of DNA synthesis when that drug is given, and are therefore shown here as the "ideal" cells for effective chemotherapy.

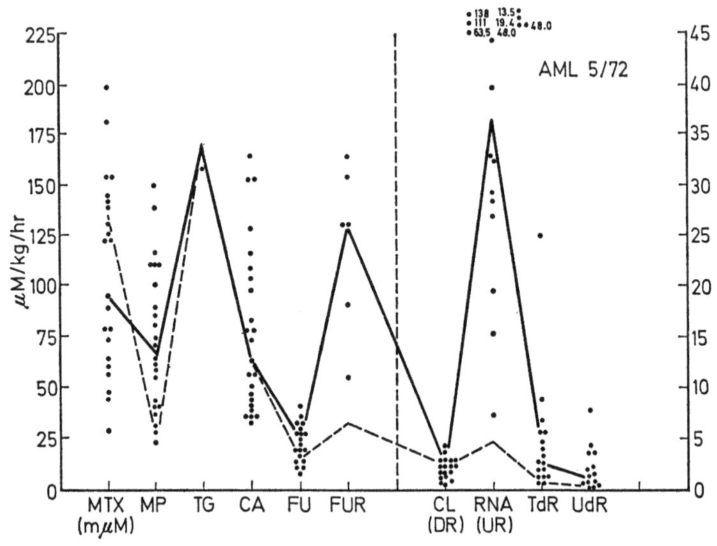

Fig. 8. Profile of blast cells from AML patients

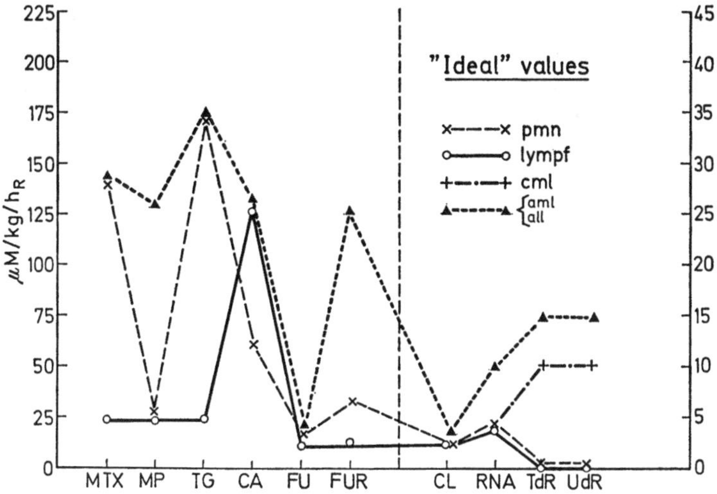

Fig. 9. Composite presentation of data from Figs. 5—8; "Ideal" values represent values found in patients later responding to, and hence "ideal" for, chemotherapy. pmn = polymorphonuclear leucocytes, lymph = normal peripheral lymphocytes, cml = mixed peripheral cells from chronic myelogenous leukemia, aml = blast cells of acute myelogenous leukemia, all = blast cells of acute lymphocytic leukemia

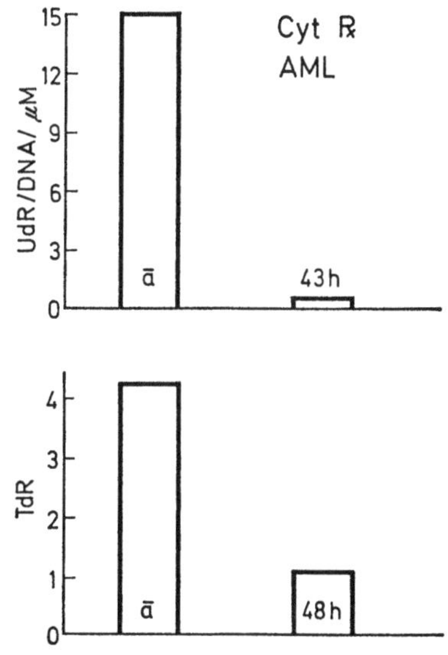

Fig. 10

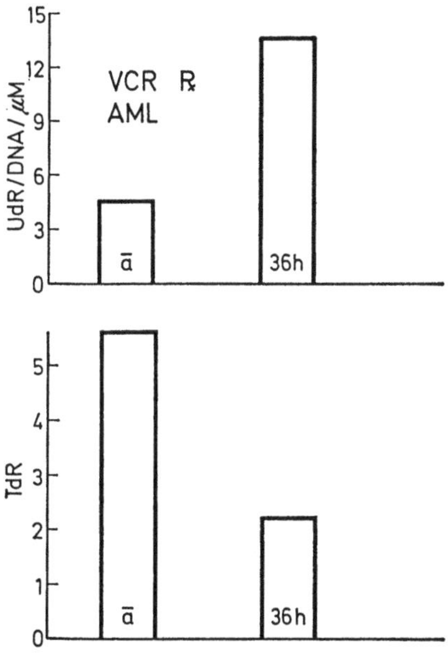

Fig. 11

In addition to the "static" biochemical morphologic picture obtained by doing one assay on a cell population, one can obtain a "dynamic" biochemical description of cell response to administration. This can be done, for example, by measuring the serial changes in DNA metabolism after a dose of test drug. Fig. 10 shows the inhibition that can be obtained with cyclophosphamide and Fig. 11 the lack of inhibition of DNA seen when a drug, e.g. Vincristine, is ineffective. We have previously published such serial changes for other drugs [7, 8].

Summary

Biochemical studies of drug responses and handling by white cells can often help to distinguish one cell type from another, or a potentially drug-sensitive leukemic blast from a resistant one. Such studies neither supplant nor diminish the role of microscopic morphology, but they can add an useful dimension to clinical therapy.

References

1. KESSEL, D., HALL, T. C.: Studies on drug transport in normal human leukocytes. Biochem. Pharmacol. **16**, 2395—2403 (1967).
2. KESSEL, D., HALL, T. C.: Retention of 6-mercaptopurine derivatives by intact cells as an index of drug response in human and murine leukemias. Cancer Res. **29**, 2116—2119 (1969).
3. GRAY, G. D., MICKELSON, M. M., HALL, T. C., KESSEL, D.: Small lymphocyte phorsphorylation of cytarabine: An organ and species survey. Biochem. Pharmacol. **21**, 2227—2236 (1972).
4. HALL, T. C., LEVINE, R.: Deamination of cytosine arabinoside by normal and malignant tissues. Proc. Amer. Ass. Cancer Res. **8**, 24 (1967).
5. HALL, T. C., KESSEL, D., LEVINE, R., ROBERTS, D.: Studies in the cellular pharmacology of cytosine arabinoside. Arzneimittel-Forsch. **19**, 20—30 (1968).
6. ROBERTS, D., HALL, T. C.: Dihydrofolate reductase activity and deoxynucleoside incorporation into DNA of human leukocytes. Cancer **20**, 905—910 (1967).
7. ROBERTS, D., HALL, T. C., ROSENTHAL, D.: Coordinated changes in thymidine 5-monophosphate metabolism of leukocytes following vincristine administration to patients with acute granulocytic leukemia. Cancer Res. **29**, 789—794 (1969).
8. ROBERTS, D., HALL, T. C., ROSENTHAL, D.: Coordinated changes in biochemical patterns: the effect of cytosine arabinoside and methotrexate on leukocytes from patients with acute granulocytic leukemia. Cancer Res. **29**, 571—578 (1969).

Conclusions of the Working Session on Nomenclature and Classification

S. PERRY

National Cancer Institute, N. I. H., Bethesda, MD/USA

I think it is fair to say that an impartial observer would have had great difficulty in coming to any conclusions as a result of the discussion concerning nomenclature and classification of the acute leukemias. The title of this session included the term workshop, which usually carries the implication that some action or recommendation will follow. However, it would be impossible for me to recommend the adoption of any set of parameters on any morphologic classification for the acute leukemias on the basis of the discussion which took place, since I am uncertain from the available information which morphologic classification and battery of measurements would be optimal. Furthermore, I doubt whether, if I were to suggest the adoption of a classification, this would be accepted by either my European or American colleagues.

Nevertheless, I firmly believe that some uniform classification is urgently needed and that Professor MATHÉ's efforts deserve support. I would suggest that a small committee be appointed, representing the EORTC and the major cooperative groups dealing with Acute Leukemia in the United States, and this Committee should devise and recommend a classification acceptable to the participating institutions.

My personal opinion is that the classification of the acute leukemias into acute lymphoid leukemia, acute myeloid leukemia, and acute monocytoid leukemia would be the least likely to evoke controversy and might be the best place to start. These broad designations are generally accepted and utilized, but I have a feeling that more detailed classifications using terms such as "prolymphoblast" and "promyeloblast" engender a good deal of resistance. The "pro" designation implies a cell somewhere between the uncommitted stem cell and the committed lymphoblast or myeloblast and I am unaware of evidence that this is a valid designation. Also there must be some provision for the range of cell types seen on most slides.

As I discussed in my presentation yesterday, the controversy over morphologic classification dates back many decades and I do not think we can put an end to it here by a vote for one or another system. Furthermore the problem of reproducibility is a serious one, and yesterday's discussion did not suggest that this has been resolved.

Moreover, morphology is a static classification and it is obvious that more than this is needed in acute leukemia. Any classification requires, it seems to me, a more dynamic assessment and the inclusion of such parameters as cytokinetic (proportion of cells in cycle, growth fraction) and cytochemical evaluation. At this point, however, the most practical course to adopt would be to include cytochemical techniques to help in discriminating among the various forms of acute leukemia. The techniques employed would of course need to be detailed and standardized.

Unfortunately, aside from morphology and cytochemical characterization, other techniques, including estimation of growth fraction, variation in cell size, etc., can and must be applied if we are to increase our knowledge about predictive factors in acute leukemia. There are many practical problems to be resolved and they need more consideration before a recommendation can be made for the universal adoption of certain techniques by the clinical groups as routine procedures.

Finally, it seems to me that there are still too many uncertainties about immunologic typing and some of the other techniques potentially useful in classification for them to be widely adopted at this time. Another problem concerns the question of the time required to perform a study. For example, in-vitro cultures and radioautography require relatively long intervals before the results are available. Hence, in a disease such as acute leukemia where the clinical course is rapid, these would be of little prospective value in any individual patient.

Thus, in summary, I recommend that 1. a committee representing the major clinical groups be established to consider the adoption of a universal classification; 2. the initial classification be a simple one; 3. along with this classification, the committee should make recommendations concerning the routine use of certain cytochemical techniques. These recommendations could then be taken into consideration by the groups concerned.

Second Session
Methodology of Clinical Trials

Introduction to Methodology of Clinical Trials in the Varieties of Acute Leukemia; Defining the Numerator and Denominator in Leukemic Trials

S. K. Carter

National Cancer Institute, N. I. H., Bethesda, MD/USA

It is common for clinicians in discussing the results of a drug trial in acute leukemia to report that the response rate is a certain %. To quote response in % assumes a numerator and a denominator figure. If the comparison of data among various groups and institutions is to be meaningful, there should be a commonly accepted definition of what constitutes the numerator and denominator for calculation of the response rates. This would appear to be a simple proposition; but in reality it can become quite complicated. An example of the difficulty is seen in Table 1; this is an abstract of an excellent paper by Bodey, Freireich *et al.* on cytosine arabinoside therapy for acute leukemia in adults. As can be seen, the authors gave a specific response figure for the drug in five different places in the text of the article. None is exactly the same, although all are valid in the terms defined.

Table 2 outlines all of the possible response rates which could be obtained from this article by utilizing the three possibilities for the numerator (CR or CR+PR or

Table 1. Cytosine arabinoside therapy for acute leukemia in adults [Bodey, Freireich *et al.* Cancer Chemother. Rep. **53**, 59—65 (1969)]

Total number of cases entered	44
Evaluable cases	36
Adequate trials	24
Complete response	9
Partial response	4
Hematologic improvement	1
Failure	10

"There were 14 responses among 36 evaluable cases." Summary, p. 59.

"The response rate for evaluable cases was 38%." Results Section, p. 60.

"The complete remission rate for those patients receiving an adequate trial (at least two courses) was 38%." Results Section, p. 60.

"The response rate for evaluable cases in this study was 39%". Discussion Section, p. 63.

"The response rate for those patients who survived long enough to receive 3 courses was 82%." Discussion Section, p. 63.

Table 2. Possible "response rates" for ARA-C therapy of AML-numerator [Bodey, Freireich *et al.* Cancer Chemother. Rep. **53**, 59—65 (1969)]

Denominator	# CR	# CR+PR	# CR+PR+HI
# Entered	9/44 (20%)	113/44 (30%)	14/44 (32%)
# Evaluable	9/36 (25%)	13/36 (36%)	14/36 (39%)
# Adequately treated	9/24 (38%)	13/24 (55%)	14/24 (60%)

CR+PR+Hl) and the three possibilities for the denominator (# entered, # evaluable, or # adequately treated). Nine possible response rates can be obtained with these variables, and the range is from a low of 20% (9 CR/44 entered) to a high of 60% (14 CR+PR+Hl/24 adequately treated). All of these nine response rates are valid calculations based on the given data. The critical problem is that no two groups present their data in exactly the same way and all, when asked, say the response rate is X %. What is needed is an agreement as to which definition will be used for both numerator and denominator in all reports of trials in leukemia.

Recently, at the National Cancer Institute, we held a conference on the current status of and future plans for acute myelocytic leukemia. Members of all the cooperative groups in the United States treating this leukemia participated and presented their latest data. It is instructive to see what numerator and denominator each group utilized, in reporting its results; an outline is given in Table 3. As can be seen, there were many differences. The National Cancer Institute had the simplest approach,

Table 3. Numerator and denominator used in AML trials of various United States groups

Group	Numerator	Denominator
National Cancer Institute	Complete remission	Number of patients
Baltimore Cancer Research Center	Complete remission	Number of patients
Acute Leukemia Group B	1. Complete remission 2. Partial remission 3. Improvement	Number of qualified or number evaluated
Southwestern Cancer Chemotherapy Cooperative Group—Study # 555	1. Complete remission 2. Improvement	1. Entered; 2. Eligible; 3. Evaluable; 4. Adequate trial
Southeastern Cancer Chemotherapy Study Group	1. Complete remission 2. Partial remission	1. Entered 2. Evaluable 3. 21 days
Western Cancer Chemotherapy Cooperative Group	1. E1 2. E2	1. Entered 2. Evaluable
Children's Cancer Study Group A	1. Complete response 2. Partial response	1. Entered 2. Adequately treated

using only one numerator (CR) and one denominator ("number of patients"). Although it is not certain whether the denominator means entered, eligible, or evaluable, etc., for other groups the possibilities went as high as six or eight for the number of "response rates" which could be elucidated from the data.

We are all familiar with the large differences reported in the literature by different groups for the results of a given drug or regimen. While patient selection and intensity schedule of therapy may be the critical variables in explaining these great differences, it is highly probable that choice of the numerator and denominator used to report the trial also plays a significant role.

Criteria for Short-Term Results in the Treatment of Acute Leukemia

G. Mathé and R. Weiner

Institut de Cancérologie et d'Immunogénétique *, Hôpital Paul-Brousse **, Villejuif/France

The aim of the treatment of acute leukemia is to cure the patient. This objective is judged by the duration of the survival of the patient and by his freedom from perceptible disease. Treatment evaluation therefore takes a long time: the actuarial curve of cumulative duration of the first remission of acute lymphoid leukemia presents as a plateau, which is the statistical expression of cure expectancy, only after 16 months (Mathé *et al.*, 1969, 1972).

As a first step in the therapeutic process, we induce a complete *remission*. We know we do not thereby eradicate the tumor cell population, we merely reduce the number of leukemic elements to a level we are not able to perceive. In so far as a complete remission is clearly defined and can be achieved in as short a time as one month or even one week, it is a *short-term result.*

For solid tumors, when they disappear after treatment, one can equally well use the words *"regression"* or remission. For acute leukemia, one has to recognize a large difference between these two terms, because acute leukemia as a syndrome comprises two diseases: a neoplasia of hematopoietic tissue, which infiltrates primarily the bone marrow and secondarily any tissue; and *bone marrow insufficiency*. The treatment can result in complete regression of the tumor with no leukemic cells detectable in any tissue, including the bone marrow, and in complete restoration of the normal hemopoietic tissue. The treatment can also result in complete regression of the tumor without restoration of the hematopoietic tissue. Only in the first instance is there an "apparently complete remission". The term "regression" more accurately describes the situation where the tumor cells disappear without hematological restoration. It nevertheless expressed the sensitivity of the tumor cells to the treatment administered.

It seems to us very important that any reports should indicate the proportion of the patients who presented a *regression without remission,* as well as those who presented a *complete remission.* It is the responsibility of all of us to distinguish clearly, in what we read as well as what we write, between "complete remission" and "complete regression". A treatment may induce a complete regression, that is the disappearance of the leukemic cells, and yet the patient may die from sustained bone marrow insufficiency. Moreover, a treatment may be excellent in terms of tumor cell

* INSERM et Association Claude-Bernard

** 14—16, av. Paul-Vaillant Couturier

Table. Proposal for the presentation of short term results

			Complete regression		Partial regression > 50%		Partial regression < 50%			Toxic cost	
Treatment	Diagnosis	Number of patients treated	With complete remission	Without complete remission	With partial remission	Without remission	With partial remission	Without remission	Failure	Lethal	Non lethal

Separate table for details

Definitions		
The tumor	Complete regression:	The disappearance of tumor cells to the limits of clinical and laboratory investigation (imperceptible disease)
	Partial regression:	The measurable reduction of tumor cells by clinical and laboratory parameters (perceptible disease)
The patient	Complete remission:	The disappearance of signs and symptoms of disease to the limits of clinical and laboratory examination of the patient
	Partial remission:	The measurable amelioration of signs and symptoms of disease by clinical and laboratory examination of the patient

regression yet too toxic for the patient, increasing hematopoietic and immune insufficiencies, and intestinal and oral mucosa lesions beyond tolerable levels.

Agents which have these drawbacks should not be rejected out of hand. Tumor cells are sensitive to them, and even if they are not able to induce remission, they may contribute beneficially to leukemia treatment if placed properly in a strategic protocol designed to eradicate the tumor cell population or reduce it to the minimal residual disease accessible to active immunotherapy. We suggest therefore that, while regressions should not be reported as remissions, they must be reported in order to let other workers know that the leukemic cells are sensitive to them.

If regressions are taken out of the realm of negative results, more reports probably will appear in the literature. For ease of reporting and especially for ease of reading and evaluating reports of therapeutic trials we propose that toxic cost be reported in the same table as the results. This will give a rapid profile of the therapy in question.

Our last remark will concern the adjective "complete": we agree that arbitrary limits of residual leukemic cells in the marrow are meaningless in terms of what we know of pharmacokinetics and of the leukemic cell load left after remission induction. We must be more strict in our morphological criteria and allow a consulting hematologist to tell us, in "blind" fashion, whether or not the bone marrow and peripheral blood are normal. If he can find no sign of abnormality on objective examination, and if the patient is clinically well, we can add the term *complete* to remission.

The Table shows the model we are currently using to present our short-term results in acute leukemia. "*Regression*" refers only to the response of the neoplasm while remission refers to the response of the *patient* in terms of all the accepted parameters.

References

MATHÉ, G., AMIEL, J. L., SCHWARZENBERG, L., SCHNEIDER, M., CATTAN, A., SCHLUMBERGER, J. R., HAYAT, M., DE VASSAL, F.: Active immunotherapy for acute lymphoid leukemia. Lancet **1969**, **1**, 697.

MATHÉ, G., POUILLART, P., SCHWARZENBERG, L., AMIEL, J. L., SCHNEIDER, M., HAYAT, M., DE VASSAL, F., JASMIN, C., ROSENFELD, C., WEINER, R., RAPPAPORT, H.: Attempts at immunotherapy of 100 acute lymphoid leukemia patients. Some factors influencing results. Nat. Cancer. Inst. Monograph, 1972, **35**, 361.

Problems in the Evaluation of Long-Term Results*

M. KARON

Division of Hematology, Department of Pediatrics, Children's Hospital of Los Angeles, and the USC School of Medicine, Los Angelos, CA/USA

Introduction

Only twelve years ago chemotherapists were struggling to increase the remission rate of children with acute lymphocytic leukemia to 50% or above and the median duration of remission to one year or more. If anyone had then expressed concern about the long-term effects of treatment or the evaluation of results, he would have been dismissed with a mild smirk and the then classical rebuff: "If someone lived long enough to develop long-term complications, we would jump for joy and treat the complications." Ironically we have now reached a time in which most of us confidently look forward to five and perhaps seven-and-a-half year median durations of survival, i.e. we are "jumping for joy", but the long-term effects of therapy and the problems of evaluating therapeutic results can no longer be easily dismissed.

A clinical trial can be conveniently divided into three segments: the front end, the middle, and the back end, each with unique implications for the evaluation of long-term results.

The Front End

Exclusion of a Poor Prognosis Group

The major problem at the front end is to discern the impact of sample heterogeneity on long-term results. The general nature of this problem is illustrated in Fig. 1. Two survival curves are shown with medians of 5 and 10 years. The two derived curves represent the hypothetical effect on the 10-year median survival of a cohort of patients whose median survival is only six months.

The striking feature of these derived data is the marked shift in the median duration of remission caused by a 10 or 20% exclusion at the front end. Additional data are given in Table 1 for several other projected medians. The calculated data in Table 1 clearly indicate that inclusion of a cohort of patients whose median duration of survival is six months or even one year, shifts the 5, 7.5 and 10-year medians in such a way as to make it impossible to carry out a comparative trial designed to detect the original difference. Clearly, if comparisons are to be made between groups,

---

* Supported by Grant CA-2649 from the National Cancer Institute, United States Public Health Service.

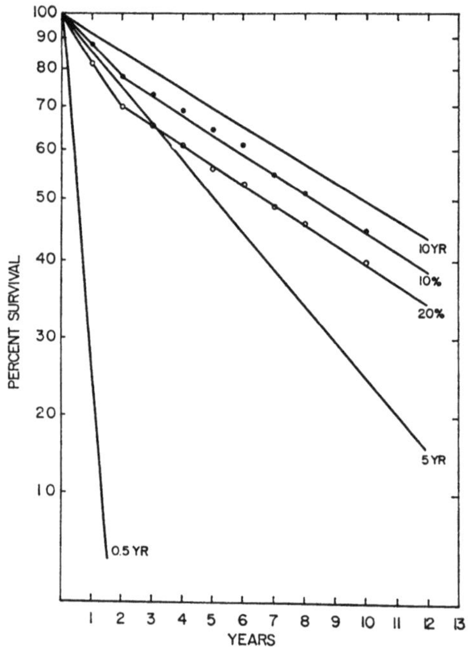

Fig. 1. Effect of a cohort of patients with a poor prognosis on the median duration of survival. The five- and ten-year survival curves are drawn assuming the exclusion of either a 10 or 20% cohort of patients who have a median survival of six months. The derived curves show the shift in median which occurs if these patients are included in the total population

the nature of the front end must be comparable in every respect, including some which we probably do not at present recognize. Such precautions are especially important when the study numbers are small.

The greater the median duration of survival projected for the clinical trial and point, the more significant is this front end problem (Fig. 2). Because small exclusions at the front end make very little difference for periods up to three years, the importance of this problem has largely gone unrecognized. This phenomenon is not necessarily restricted to exclusions or induction failures; it can also obtain for any cohort of patients with a certain set of disease characteristics that result in a survival pattern significantly different from that of the rest of the population.

Table 1. Front end exclusion vs. median duration

Expected median	Cohort median	Calculated median (yr)	
		10%	20%
2	0.5	1.8	1.6
5	0.5	4.3	3.5
	1.0	4.3	3.4
7.5	0.5	6.2	5.0
10	0.5	8.0	6.7

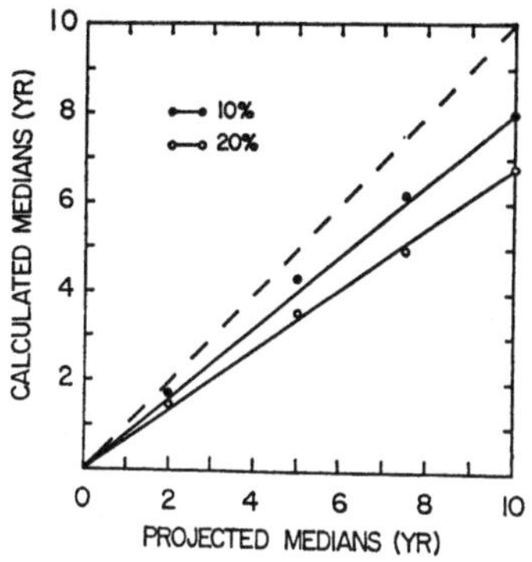

Fig. 2. Relationship of the projected medians to the medians derived by including the poor prognostic cohorts. The derived curves show the effect on projected medians at 2, 5, 7.5 and 10 years of the inclusion of a cohort of patients with a median survival of six months representing either 10 or 20% of the total population

Evidence for Cohorts with Distinct Prognostic Characteristics

One of the better-studied prognosticators is the initial white blood cell count [3, 4]. The interpretive dilemma that can arise out of this problem is illustrated in Fig. 3, which represents data comparing five treatment regimens for remission maintenance, taken from a recent study under the chairmanship of Dr. Denis Miller of the Children's Cancer Study Group A. This study developed no significant difference in the median duration of remission. A significant difference, however, could be observed if one were to analyze the duration of remission in terms of three ranges of initial white blood cell counts. In spite of the statistical analysis, one has an uneasy feeling that differences in the effect of therapy might have been obscured.

Table 2. Defining the problems at the front end

Cytology
Morphology—histochemistry
Membrane antigens or antibodies
Cytogenetics
Age
Tumor distribution
CNS
Organs
Growth rate
WBC
Uric acid
Macromolecular synthesis
Marrow function
Pressure and flow
"Stem" cell culture
Immune status

The initial white blood cell count is clearly not the only factor which can be used to identify sub-populations. A more complete outline is given in Table 2. Morphology has prognostic implications [4]. With more subtle techniques, many of which have been discussed at this meeting, important morphological subclassifications in acute lymphocytic leukemia may assume prognostic significance. Age has prognostic significance in every childhood tumor system investigated to date, and leukemia is no exception [3]. The distribution and degree of leukemic infiltration has recently been shown to be an important prognosticator [2]. Better estimates of the growth rate of leukemia cells and more sophisticated measurements of bone marrow function may also provide information which could be used to identify prognostic subcategories. The measurement of the immune status has important prognostic implications in acute myelogenous leukemia, and needs to be investigated in acute lymphocytic leukemia [5].

Problems in the Middle

The problems encountered during the maintenance part of a study that have implications for long-term evaluation are listed in Table 3. Long-term results are most likely to be significant if the child remains in initial remission for over 90% of treatment time. Patients who relapse from the primary regimen will ordinarily be treated with drugs which have less probability of maintaining remission. The development of

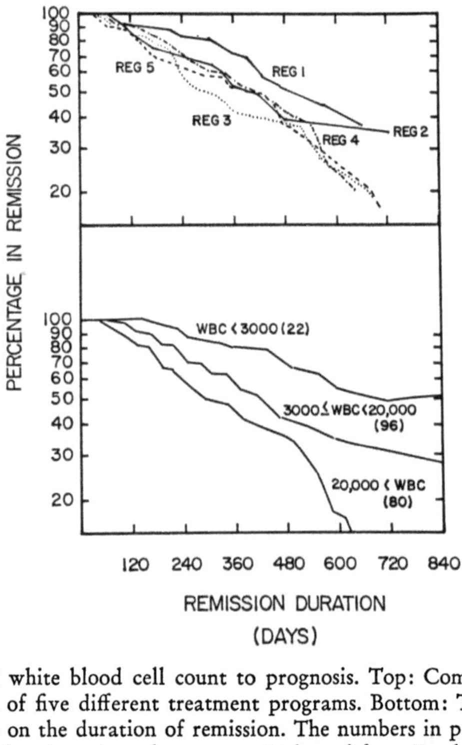

Fig. 3. Relationship of white blood cell count to prognosis. Top: Comparison of the median durations of remission of five different treatment programs. Bottom: The effect of the initial white blood cell count on the duration of remission. The numbers in parenthesis represent the number of patients in each category. (Adapted from Breslow, 1972)

newer, more effective drugs and their use in combination with older agents can change this process and form the basis for projecting continued improvement in survival [7]. Such developments can also change the interpretation of the importance of the initial remission in evaluating the total survival experience.

Table 3. Problems in the middle

Relapse
Bone marrow
CNS
Other
Death in remission
Related to therapy
Unrelated
Toxicity

End Points

The "maintenance" phase can end in one of three ways: relapse in bone marrow, CNS or other extramedullary site; death in remission from causes related or unrelated to treatment; or toxicity requiring the discontinuance of therapy. Each of these three end points needs to be analyzed separately as a function of time. All too frequently such information is "lumped" into a remission maintenance curve, thus throwing away valuable information for predicting the toxic cost of treatment and the biology of extramedullary relapse.

Meningeal Leukemia

Meningeal infiltration in leukemia has long been considered a potential source for generating relapse in the bone marrow. If this hypothesis is correct, control of CNS leukemia should result in an increase in the duration of remission. A study begun in 1963 by Acute Leukemia Group B, using prophylactic intrathecal methotrexate, reduced the incidence of meningeal leukemia but failed to demonstrate any prolongation of remission [3] (Table 4). On the other hand, a later study by the same Group

Table 4. Prophylactic I. T. MTX vs. duration of remission

Study	Year	I. T. methotrexate	No. patients	% meningeal leukemia	Remission duration (months)
Frei *et al.*	1963	None	34	24	7
		Monthly	35	3	7
Holland *et al.*	1968	None	116	30—40	15
		Weekly-monthly ×6	117	< 10	26

indicated that prophylactic intrathecal methotrexate not only reduces the incidence of meningeal leukemia but can also prolong remission [6]. The most striking difference between these two studies is in the median duration of remission: 7 months in the earlier study against 15 or 26 months in the latter. Since the incidence of meningeal leukemia is a function of time, the effect of prophylactic intrathecal methotrexate was probably not demonstrable when the duration of bone marrow remission was short. These findings emphasize the importance of the time parameter for the assessment of each end point in the maintenance phase of a study.

Problems at the Back End

The main problems at the back end of a clinical trial are tabulated in Table 5.

Table 5. Problems at the back end

Evaluating survival
Quality of life
Reinduction vs. recurrence
Long-term follow-up

Evaluation

One of the most difficult tasks in the evaluation of long-term results is the recognition of a significantly different treatment result in the shortest possible time following the close of a particular study. Heretofore, this period has been in the neighborhood of three to five years, a relatively workable time for evaluating the back end of a comparative trial.

A nice illustration of the magnitude of the problems is given in Table 6. These projections are based on the assumption that the present yearly rate of increase in the median duration of survival of children with acute lymphocytic leukemia obeys a log-normal distribution and can be projected from the solid data base of Acute Leukemia Group B [7]. For a two- or three-arm study, requiring approximately 102 patients per arm to evaluate a projected 50% difference in medians, the time required to collect enough patients will be two years. The time required to evaluate the study from the last patient entry is estimated to be approximately one year longer than the longest median duration, but it could be longer. Such a projection is probably not far from the truth, and it predicts that the ability to distinguish between survival for 7.5 and for 10 years would occur in 1991.

This long period of time, 19 years, has major implications for the evaluation of results. Mechanisms for long-term follow-up and maintenance of study discipline need to be sharpened, and must allow for the mobility of the population and have the capability of ferreting out late complications, especially the cause of death. The typical child of 5 may require 40 to 50 years of follow-up to determine "cure" and the true impact of therapy.

Table 6. Projection. Age of investigator vs. duration of study

Proposed survival difference	Estimated [a] year of diagnosis	Study time		Total (yr)	Year of answer
		Accrual	Evaluation (yr)		
5	1972	2	8	10	1982
7.5	1975	2	8	10	1985
7.5	1975	2	11	13	1988
10	1978	2	11	13	1991

[a] Log Normal Distribution (LINCOLN and WELLS, 1972) used to predict the year of diagnosis for the projected survival differences based on the current status of the art.

Quality of Life

Those who treat acute lymphocytic leukemia long ago established the fact that the child in remission is a well child. The short-term side effects of cytotoxic agents are counterbalanced by a relatively longer period of good health. The quality of life for a long-term survivor, however, is more related to his subsequent ability to cope in the adult world. A primary concern here is the effect of therapy on fertility, teratogenesis and carcinogenesis. Although these are matters which are rather difficult to monitor, they may ultimately be the determinants of whether a particular treatment program initiated in childhood is as good as an alternate therapy.

Recurrence vs. Induction

The question whether late recurrent disease represents a new tumor clone has always been moot in the absence of a significant number of long-term survivors. The recent observations from laboratories performing bone marrow transplantation, indicating that leukemia can occur in donor cells [8], have heightened interest in the resolution of this question. There are several possible approaches, involving cytogenetic markers, membrane antigens and antibodies, morphological and histological criteria, isoenzymes, virological studies, etc. Of primary importance is that the problem be recognized and appropriate materials be obtained at the front end of the study program.

Conclusion

The main difficulty in the evaluation of long-term results is the time required to tell whether one treatment program is significantly different from another. The longer the duration of survival, the more likely is the median to be profoundly affected by a variety of factors, especially those which can occur at the front end. Even with conservative estimates, it is quite clear that the time required to evaluate such studies will be longer than the lifetime of some of the investigators now involved in such programs. It is imperative, therefore, that consideration be given to alternative approaches as well as to setting up systems for long-term follow-up of these valuable patients.

One alternative approach is to try harder at the front end and middle of a clinical trial to identify those factors which are of prognostic significance, and then design new therapeutic programs for patients whose survival characteristics are significantly worse than those of the group as a whole. The time required to collect enough patients for a comparative trial of the effect of several regimens on long-term survival is now so long that four to five additional studies need to be mounted before the result of the initial program is available. This phenomenon suggests that future progress is more likely to occur at the front end and middle of a clinical trial, where the assessment of new therapies can be made in a reasonable time, and that future increases in survival will be a byproduct and not the consequence of analysis of the back end of the treatment result.

References

1. BRESLOW, N.: Covariance analysis of censored survival data. 1972 (in press).
2. FITZPATRICK, J., LIEBERMAN, N., SINKS, L. F.: A comparative study of CNS involvement in childhood lymphosarcoma. Boston: ASCO 1972.
3. FREI, E., KARON, M., LEVIN, R. H., FREIREICH, E. J., TAYLOR, R. J., HANANIAN, J., SELAWRY, O., HOLLAND, J. F., HOOGSTRATEN, B., WOLMAN, I. J., ESSHAGH, A., SAWITSKY, A., LEE, S., MILLS, S. D., BURGERT, E. O., SPURR, C. L., PATTERSON, R. B., EBAUGH, F. G., JAMES, G. W., MOON, J. H.: The effectiveness of combinations of antileukemic agents in inducing and maintaining remission in children with acute leukemia. Blood **26**, 642 (1965).
4. FREIREICH, E. J., GEHAN, E. A., SULMAN, P., BOGGS, D. R., FREI, E.: The effect of chemotherapy on acute leukemia in the human. J. chron. Dis. **14**, 593 (1961).
5. HERSH, E. M., WHITECAR, J. P., MCCREDIE, K. B., BODEY, G. P., FREIREICH, E. J.: Acute leukemia: Therapy, immunocompetence, immunosuppression and prognosis. New Engl. J. Med. **285**, 1211 (1971).
6. HOLLAND, J.: This symposium. 1972.
7. LINCOLN, T. L., WELLS, R. E.: Predicting progress, recognizing breakthroughs, and evaluating performance in the treatment of leukemia. J. Math. Bioscience 1972 (in press).
8. THOMAS, E. D., BUCKNER, C. D., FEFER, A., NEIMAN, P., BRYANT, J. I., CLIFT, R. A., JOHNSON, F. L., RAMBERG, R. E., STORB, R.: Leukemic transformation of ingrafted human marrow cells in vivo. Lancet **1972** (in press).

Attempts at Standardization of Methods and Expression of Results

D. E. Bergsagel and D. H. Cowan

Princess Margaret Hospital, Toronto/Canada and Department of Medicine, Princess Margaret Hospital and the Ontario Cancer Institute, and Sunnybrook Hospital and the University of Toronto, Toronto/Canada

Introduction

Methods of conducting clinical trials must be similar, so that different centers can make general comparisons of the results of their approaches to treatment. The factors that need to be standardized for these comparisons include the criteria for selecting or excluding leukemic patients, and the criteria used in the evaluation of short- and long-term results. These aspects have been considered by Drs. Frei, Freireich and Karon. In this paper we consider the expression of the results of clinical trials in the treatment of acute leukemia.

We doubt that it would be advisable to devise standardized methods for expressing the results of clinical trials, because each trial is an experiment, and the methods used to analyse the results will vary depending on the questions that are asked. For this reason, we will not outline a dogmatic program for the assessment of results. Instead, we will consider some of the factors which have been found to be valuable in the analysis of previous clinical trials, while fully realizing that important questions, such as those related to the mechanisms involved in the induction of remission and relapse, have not been posed or investigated. The factors that are now known to be useful in the analysis of results are: the frequency of complete remissions; the duration of the remissions; the survival of patients; comparisons of the responder and failure groups; and the toxic cost to patients. Each of these factors will be considered. The examples used to illustrate some of these points are based on the results of treating a group of adult patients with acute myeloblastic leukemia, reported by Abu-Zahra, Clarysse, Cowan, Hasselback and Bergsagel (1972).

Frequency of Complete Remissions

As Freireich and Frei (1964) have noted, the induction of a complete remission is the most important event in acute leukemia. However, we must remember that the reported frequency of complete remissions is greatly influenced by the denominator which is selected. Many investigators believe that the most significant figure is the percentage of all patients started on a treatment program who achieve a complete remission. Others feel that the group of patients who receive inadequate treatment because therapy was stopped for reasons other than failure, or because of early death of the patient, should be subtracted from the denominator. Since there are good reasons to support both of these views, we believe it is necessary to report all of the data shown in Table 1.

Table 1. Acute leukemia — Frequency of complete remissions

1. Number started on treatment protocol.
2. Inadequate treatment:
a. Therapy stopped for reasons other than failure.
b. Early death.
3. Complete remissions:
a. % of 1
b. % of (1 minus 2)
c. % of (1 minus 2 a)

Duration of Complete Remission

Since the duration of the remission is the most important factor influencing the survival of patients with acute leukemia (Freireich, Gehan, Sulman, Boggs and Frei, 1961), this aspect of the results must be considered (Table 2). The duration of the remission following discontinuation of all therapy makes it possible to estimate the residual number of leukemic cells (Frei and Freireich, 1965), and reports of the site of leukemic relapse may suggest additional therapeutic measures, such as radiation of the cranium combined with intrathecal, methotrexate (Aur, Hustu, Verzosa, Wood and Simone, 1972), for prolonging the duration of the remission. An analysis of chromosome markers in leukemic cells prior to treatment and after relapse is of considerable value in determining whether the relapse is due to regrowth of the original leukemic stem line, (Reisman, Mitani and Zuelzer, 1964; Hart, Trujillo, Freireich, George and Frei, 1971) or the induction of leukemia in a new stem line (Fialkow, Thomas, Bryant and Neiman, 1971).

Table 2. Acute leukemia — Duration of complete remission

1. On maintenance therapy.
2. After stopping therapy.
3. Site of relapse (compare chromosome marker with pretreatment).
a. Marrow
b. CNS
c. Other

Survival

The influence of treatment on the survival of patients is considered to be the most important measurement of the effect of treatment on the leukemic process. When the patients entered on a clinical trial are a mixture of previously treated and previously untreated patients, the survival from diagnosis is difficult to interpret because this figure is unduly influenced by the selected group of previously treated patients who have lived long enough to be entered into the new treatment protocol (Fig. 1). Survival from the onset of the new treatment is a much more meaningful figure, for the survival of previously treated and previously untreated patients is usually very similar when it is measured from the onset of the treatment protocol (Fig. 2).

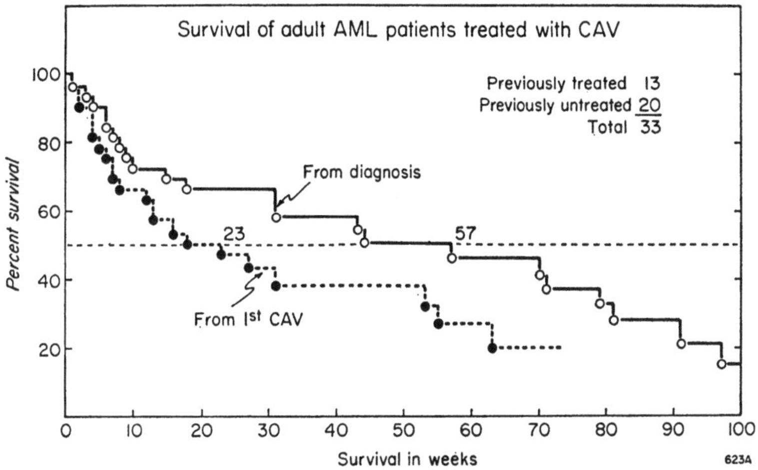

Fig. 1. Survival of 33 adult patients with acute myeloblastic leukemia is plotted in weeks from diagnosis, and from the start of cyclophosphamide, arabinosyl cytosine and vincristine (CAV) treatment. The median survival in weeks is indicated for both survival curves

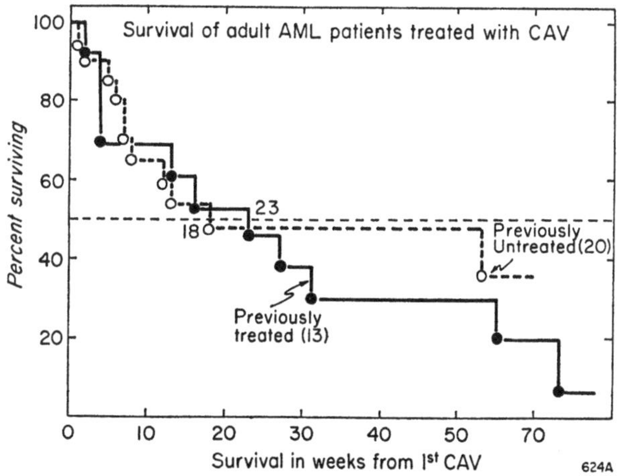

Fig. 2. Survival of 20 previously untreated, and 13 previously treated patients with acute myeloblastic leukemia is plotted in weeks from the start of cyclophosphamide, arabinosyl cytosine and vincristine (CAV). The median survival in weeks for both groups is indicated

Comparison of Responders and Failures

A comparison of some features of the patients who fail with those who achieve a complete remission is of considerable interest (Table 3). For example, as many other investigators have noted, the age of the leukemic patient has a very important influence on his chances of achieving a complete remission. In the example shown in this Table, the probability of patients under the age of 38 achieving a complete remission was 12/16 (75%) while for those over 38 the probability was only 3/14 (21%). The difference between these remission rates is highly significant ($p = 0.004$). The group was divided at age 38, because the median age for all patients was 37.6 years.

Table 3. Adult AML treated with CAV[a]: Responders vs. failures

	Responders		Failures
Number	15		15
Age (yrs) median (range)	32 (17—55)		44 (19—60)
<38	12		4
		p=0.004	
>38	3		11
Media survival (weeks)			
from 1st CAV	63		7
less time in CR	16		—

[a] A combination of cyclophosphamide, arabinosyl cytosine and vincristine.

Although the time spent in complete remission is the most important factor influencing the improved survival of the responder group (Freireich *et al.*, 1961), the fact that the median survival time of the responders, after subtracting the time spent in complete remission, is 9 weeks longer than the median survival of the nonresponder suggests that factors other than the duration of the complete remission probably influence the survival of these two groups of patients.

Toxic Cost to the Patient

When one attempts to evaluate whether a particular form of treatment is beneficial to a patient, one must consider the toxic cost to the patient. This can be done in many ways, for example, by enumerating the number of days of fever, the duration of leukopenia and thrombocytopenia, or the cost to the patient of hospitalization, drugs and other services. Abu-Zahra *et al.* (1972), chose to evaluate the cost to the patient in terms of the percentage of time spent in hospital after the diagnosis of acute leukemia, and compared this with the duration of survival. They found that patients who fail to achieve a complete remission spent over 80% of their time in hospital. In contrast, the percentage of the patients' total survival time in hospital declined gradually for the patients who achieved complete remissions, until a plateau of 25% was reached at about 150 days.

The methods I have presented for the expression of results of clinical trials in acute leukemia are relatively standard. These methods are quite useful for analysing the results of clinical trials designed to answer the questions which we have learned how to pose. The methods will have to change as we learn how to ask more intelligent and pertinent questions.

References

ABU-ZAHRA, H., CLARYSSE, A., COWAN, D. H., HASSELBACK, R., BERGSAGEL, D. E.: Treatment of acute myeloblastic leukemia in adults: remission induction with a combination of cyclophosphamide, arabinosyl cytosine and vincristine (CAV). Submitted to Canad. med. Ass. J.

AUR, R., HUSTU, H., VERZOSA, M., WOOD, A., SIMONE, J.: Two forms of "prophylactic" central nervous system therapy in childhood acute lymphocytic leukemia. Proc. Amer. Ass. Cancer Res. **13**, 54 (1972).

FIALKOW, P. J., THOMAS, E. D., BRYANT, J. I., NEIMAN, P. E.: Leukaemic transformation of engrafted human marrow cells *in vivo*. Lancet **1971 I**, 255.

FREI, E. III., FREIREICH, E. J.: Progress and perspectives in the chemotherapy of acute leukemia. Advanc. Chemother. **2**, 269 (1965).

FREIREICH, E. J., FREI, E. III.: Recent advances in acute leukemia. Progr. Hemat. **4**, 187 (1964).

FREIREICH, E. J., GEHAN, E. A., SULMAN, D., BOGGS, D. R., FREI, E. III.: The effects of chemotherapy on acute leukemia in the human J. chron. Dis. **14**, 593 (1961).

HART, J. S., TRUJILLO, J. M., FREIREICH, E. J., GEORGE, S. L., FREI, E. III.: Cytogenetic studies and their clinical correlates in adults with acute leukemia. Ann. int. Med. **75**, 353 (1971).

REISMAN, L. E., MITANI, M., ZUELZER, W. W.: Chromosome studies in leukemia. New Engl. J. Med. **270**, 591 (1964).

The Analysis of Clinical Trials in Leukaemia

M. C. Pike

DHSS Cancer Epidemiology and Clinical Trials Unit, Department of the Regius, Oxford University, Oxford/England

Three related questions which have been discussed at this meeting fall within the fields of epidemiology and medical statistics. These questions are:

1. Why does the "same" protocol produce different results at different centres?
2. How should the results of clinical trials be presented (published)?
3. What statistical methods should be used in the analysis of trial results?

It has always appeared to me that to make one's point in discussing such questions a certain amount of exaggeration is desirable. I will follow this rule.

DOGMA 1 — It is a Waste of Time to Compare Results in Different Centres

It is generally accepted that without comparability of referral pattern to different centres there is no reason to expect comparability of results, and experience of listening to discussions of this question of referral pattern at meeting after meeting will certainly have convinced all of us that it is a sterile subject for discussion. This is one reason why Dogma 1 is nearly true.

Known facts concerning the epidemiology of acute lymphoblastic leukaemia (ALL) in children illustrate a second reason, viz. that leukaemia may not be the same disease from one place to another. Firstly, diagnosis of leukemia varies widely from place to place (Stewart and Barber, 1971), so that even if all cases in an area are accepted by a centre the cases will be different from place to place as some cases in one area would not have been diagnosed in another. Secondly, and more importantly, we now have good evidence that maternal irradiation (Stewart and Barber, 1971) and probably maternal influenza and varicella infection (Adelstein and Donovan, 1972; Bithell, Draper and Gorbach, 1972; Fedrick and Alberman, 1972) "cause" ALL in some children—is this "ordinary" ALL in treatment terms? It is unlikely to be so in all respects. The results of the Memphis group, showing that Negro children with ALL have a worse prognosis than white children, also bear this out (Walters, Bushore and Simone, 1972). So the "sort" of leukaemia and the "sort" of host are going to change with time and place.

It is for these reasons, as well as some others, that one does randomized clinical trials instead of the much simpler and quicker historical comparisons. It is surely illogical of us to randomize in our own current trial while expecting to be able to make valid between-centre or between-continent comparisons.

It is, of course, obligatory on clinicians to try to understand how the current "best" results are being obtained—for example, maybe the strictness with which the treatment schedule is adhered to has a great effect—but if comparability, after allowing for known prognostic factors, cannot be obtained, it does not necessarily mean that either party is somehow misreporting.

DOGMA 2 — You Haven't Analysed Your Results Enough

The cost of treating each patient in a leukaemia trial must be well in excess of £ 1000. An "average" trial will have say 100 patients entered so we are talking in terms of £ 100,000 or more. With this in mind very few trials have the short of care devoted to their analysis that they warrant. A small increase in information gleaned by thorough analysis should amply repay the effort involved.

The recent analysis of the UK Medical Research Council's (MRC) first trial in myelomatosis illustrate this (MRC, 1972). Table 1 gives the observed (O) and expected (E) number of deaths in this trial (as of 1 March 1972) according to the blood urea of the patients at presentation (see below for method of calculating E). It can be seen from the column O/E that the lower the initial blood urea the better the prognosis. This is a well-known effect, but further analysis brought to light an entirely new prognostic factor, viz. serum albumin (Table 2). Table 3 investigates these two factors simultaneously and shows that they are essentially independent. This has directed laboratory workers to a new and hopefully fruitful aspect of myeloma cell metabolism.

Detailed analysis should also lead to a fuller understanding of what the treatment is accomplishing. For example, in the MRC trial of BCG for the maintenance treatment of ALL after 5 months of "intensive" therapy, the results shown in Table 4 were obtained (up to 1 March 1972). These appear to imply that the BCG did not work and that the intermittent methotrexate did. But that is less than half the story.

Table 1. UK MRC first myelomatosis trial. Survival from first treatment

Blood urea at presentation (mg/100 ml)	N, no. of patients in group	O, observed no. of deaths	E, expected no. of deaths	Relative death rate, O/E
0–	113	79	122.1	0.65
40–	92	81	74.6	1.09
80+	53	53	16.3	3.24
All	258	213	213.0	1.00

Table 2. UK MRC first myelomatosis trial. Survival from first treatment

Serum albumin at presentation (g/100 ml)	N, no. of patients in group	O, observed no. of deaths	E, expected no. of deaths	Relative death rate, O/E
0.0–	44	42	22.8	1.84
3.0–	125	105	96.3	1.09
4.0+	89	66	93.9	0.70
All	258	213	213.0	1.00

Table 3. UK MRC first myelomatosis trial. Survival from first treatment

Blood urea at presentation (mg/100 ml)	Serum albumin at presentation (g/100 ml) [a]			
	0.0–	3.0–	4.0+	All
0–	15/14/10.5 1.33	54/41/53.0 0.77	44/24/58.5 0.41	113/79/122.1 0.65
40–	17/16/9.1 1.76	45/38/37.4 1.02	30/27/28.1 0.96	92/81/74.6 1.09
80+	12/12/3.2 3.75	26/26/5.9 4.44	15/15/7.3 2.06	53/53/16.3 3.24
All	44/42/22.8 1.84	125/105/96.3 1.09	89/66/93.9 0.70	258/213/213.0 1.00

[a] Data are given as: N/O/E
O ÷ E
where N = no. of patients in group
O = observed number of deaths in group
E = expected number of deaths in group
O ÷ E = relative death rate in group

Table 4. UK MRC BCG trial in acute lymphoblastic leukaemia. Remission after randomisation

Maintenance treatment	N, no. of patients in group	O, observed no. of first relapses	E, expected no. of first relapses	Relative relapse rate, O/E
Methotrexate	53	35	54.4	0.64
BCG	51	46	33.7	1.37
None	18	17	9.9	1.72
All	122	98	98.0	1.00

Table 5. UK MRC BCG trial in acute lymphoblastic leukaemia. Remission after randomisation

Leucocyte count at presentation (/ml)	Treatment [a]			
	Methotrexate	BCG	None	All
0–	24/11/31.8 0.35	21/16/17.6 0.91	6/6/2.9 2.09	51/33/52.3 0.63
6000–	14/11/14.7 0.75	15/15/8.6 1.74	6/6/5.0 1.21	35/32/28.3 1.13
21000+	15/13/7.9 1.64	15/15/7.4 2.02	6/5/2.0 2.45	36/33/17.4 1.90
All	53/35/54.4 0.64	51/46/33.7 1.37	18/17/9.9 1.72	122/98/98.0 1.00

[a] Data are given as: N/O/E
O ÷ E
where N = no. of patients in group
O = observed no. of first relapses in group
E = expected no. of first relapses in group
O ÷ E = relative first relapse rate in group

Table 5 shows first that the leukocyte count *on admission* is still of major prognostic importance when the patient is in complete remission five months later. Secondly, for the patients who originally presented with low leukocyte counts there is some evidence that BCG had an effect. This suggests, in agreement with animal work, that further attempts at immunotherapy should initially be concentrated on patients with good prognosis. Thirdly, maintenance methotrexate therapy as given in this trial does little or nothing to prolong the first remission of those who present with a high leukocyte count, and that a new approach needs to be adopted to maintenance treatment protocols for these high-risk patients.

DOGMA 3 — Report Your Results in the Greatest Detail

Subject to the well-known fact that the number of readers of a paper is inversely proportional to its length, report your results in the greatest detail. Furthermore, if you want me to read it, then note that I only read summaries, tables and look at figures. If I get the wrong message from these then it is the author's fault. Conveying information in this manner may annoy editors who prefer text to tables and figures but the reality of my, and most readers, behaviour must be allowed to be paramount.

We have been offered a long string of things to report: No. Entered, No. Evaluable, No. Adequately treated, No. CR, No. CR or PR, No. CR or PR or HI.

It is only really necessary to have all this variety if the different parameters tell a different story. For example, an "intense" regime may kill a lot of patients through making them, say, very susceptible to infection, but if they survive the intensive phase they do much better. In a centre with "poor" facilities the regime may not look good overall, but very good duration of remission in the adequately treated would make it ethical to test the regime if much greater supportive care, such as life-islands, could be provided.

It would also help if "Adequately treated" (and the like) was defined precisely in time terms, e.g. "Adequately treated" as alive at 6 weeks. In my experience, PR and HI very seldom contain any extra information and should be dropped.

DOGMA 4 — Use "Logrank" Scores to Analyse the Results

Standard actuarial survival curves (or remission duration curves) provide the most accurate summary of survival time date. These should be plotted with the vertical "% survivors" axis on a logarithmic scale, so that the slope of the curve at any given time estimates the "death" rate at that time: points for individual patients should be given whenever possible, so that the number of cases the curve is based on at any given time can readily be seen.

Tests of significance between groups of survival times should be performed by the Logrank test (described in the Appendix)—this test is optimum in that, if differences between groups exist, then the test is more likely to detect the differences than any other test. It can be used for comparisons of multiple groups of patients, with the groups being defined not only by treatment schedule but by any factor that may be of prognostic importance (see Tables 1—5). It has the added advantages of being easy to use, once grasped, and of being non-parametric, that is, it does not assume that the survival (or remission duration) curves follow any particular distribution, such as log-normal or exponential.

DOGMA 5 — Think (Biologically)

Even the best statistical test is of little value unless applied with considerable thought. For example, if we are comparing a "mild" and a "severe" regime then the "mild" one may appear better if we look at the proportion survivors at 1 year but worse if we look at the proportion survivors at 5 years. Most statistical tests (including the Logrank test) will in these circumstances favour the "mild" regime (Mantel, 1966) so if we are really interested in the "long term" survivors we need to match our test to the question. Similarly a "mild" regime may be better than a "severe" one for "good prognosis" patients but worse for "bad prognosis" patients; this would be a critical observation and no statistical test can be expected to seek for this on its own.

Generally speaking, leukemia trials have concentrated up to now on the problem of finding the most effective treatment regime for general recommendation, with correspondingly less attention being given to investigating individual patient's response to their disease. We are accustomed to modifying drug dosages depending on the haematological response; we should now concentrate more attention on extending this. By monitoring the individual patient's progress by clinical and laboratory methods, it may be possible to adjust the treatment with some precision according to the individual's own "needs". Clinical trials will then be designed to test one "treatment concept" against another rather than one "drug regime" against another, that is, we will test flexible regimes in which the treatment is *radically* varied depending on variables which are continuously measured in the individual patient.

DOGMA 6 — An Ethical Comparative Trial Can only be Done by Remaining Ignorant of the Intermediate Results

Suppose 40 patients have been entered in a comparative trial of two drug schedules A and B, 20 on each schedule; and that individual results can be expressed soon after administration of the treatment as "good" or "bad" and that they are as follows:

	"Good"	"Bad"	Total
A	16	4	20
B	9	11	20

This distribution is not quite significant at the 5% level. Public ethics or the ethics of the long-term good tell us to go on and randomly allocate the next patient to A or B. But I doubt whether any physician would behave this way, since he is trained to act in the light of private ethics, or doing what looks like the best for the patient now in front of him. He must opt for A. He can avoid the conflict only by remaining in ignorance of the intermediate results. (The trial results need, of course, to be kept under constant surveillance by someone not actually treating the patients.)

This is *not* an argument for abandoning clinical trials, but rather to make the point that public ethics must of necessity have a paramount position in any discussion of trials. Concepts such as "informed consent" do not really allow us to avoid the issue.

DOGMA 7 — Do Your Trials Quickly

This Dogma is closely related to Dogma 6.

Before a trial has gone on very long, stories of marvellous results from other trials will make it very difficult, if not unethical, for physicians not to want to change at least some of the treatment protocol. Therefore, to offer the best chance of getting enough data together to be meaningful before the pressure to change schedules becomes overwhelming, trials should preferably have only two treatment groups.

To sum up: For ethical and scientific reasons at lot of time should be spent deciding what question the trial is to answer, bearing in mind the rate of entry of patients to the trial; without a good question, the trial is by definition bad. Then analyse the results of a sensible question trial in great detail, report them in full and do not be completely thrown off balance, if when comparing them to other trial results, they do not appear quite so good.

Statistical Appendix

The Logrank Method of Analysing "Survival Times"

The standard actuarial technique fo· calculating remission duration curves can be described as follows: Consider a group of patients who have achieved remission and have been followed up to some date. By this date, some patients will have relapsed with differing first remission durations and other will still be in their first remission with remission durations therefore known to be in excess of certain times. Their observed relapse rate on a particular day after entering remission, say day 82, is the proportion of those patients who, still in first remission at the end of the first 81 days, relapsed on the 82nd day. Write this as q_{82} and write $p_{82} = 1 - q_{82}$. Now the proportion of patients still in remission at the end of, for example, day 96 after entering remission is estimated actuarially by $p_1 * p_2 * \ldots * p_{96}$. The remission length life-table is a table or graph of this estimate against time from entering remission. It can be proved to be the most accurate summary of the data.

Treatment differences between two groups of patients is first investigated visually by calculating and plotting their separate life-tables. The statistical significance of any observed difference between these life-tables of the two treatment groups is assessed by first giving each patient a score expressing how well he has done and then evaluating by standard randomization methods the statistical significance of the difference between the average scores in the two groups.

A scoring system with very good statistical properties and which is also obviously sensible can be described as follows: suppose at the end of day 81 from start of treatment there are *in both groups combined* 16 patients still in remission and being observed through day 82. Suppose further that 2 of them relapse on day 82 so that $q_{82} = 2/16 = 0.125$. Each of these 16 patients may be thought of as having had a "hazard" to face of this amount, q_{82}. A patient who is still in remission with a remission time to date of T has faced successively the hazards q_1, q_2, up to q_T. His score is taken to be the sum of these, viz. ($q_1 + \ldots + q_T$). A patient who relapses at time T has faced the same total of hazards but his score is decreased by 1 for the fact of his relapse; thus his score is $(q_1 + \ldots + q_T) - 1$. This may be written as $U = (q_1 + \ldots + q_T) - d$, where $d=1$ if the patient has relapsed, and $d=0$ otherwise. $e=(q_1+\ldots+q_T)$ may conveniently be thought of as the patient's "expected relapse" so that the patient's score, $U=e-d$ is the difference between his "expected" and "observed" relapse.

One then finds the expected, E, and observed, O, number of relapses for each of the two groups of patients by summing the individual *e's* and *d's*. E for a group is equal to the number of relapses that one would expect to have found in that group, *after allowing for the durations of their exposure to risk, and if the prognosis of that group is the same as that of the other group.* The ratio O/E for a group is called the relative relapse rate, because it equals the ratio of the average relapse rate in that group to the overall average relapse rate.

The approximate statistical significance of any difference in observed, O, and expected, E, deaths in the two groups can be rapidly found by summing $(O-E)^2/E$ over both groups and regarding this as a chi-squared distribution on 1 degree of freedom (PETO and PETO, 1972). To calculate more precise significance levels is simple but tedious—see MANTEL (1966) and COX (1972) for details.

The statistical test based on these observed and expected numbers of relapses can be shown, for the usual clinical trial situations, to be optimum in the sense that if one protocol is better than the other then no other statistical test is more likely to detect this difference (PETO and PETO, 1972).

These methods can be extended to the comparison of more than two groups of patients and also to allow for explanatory information, e.g. initial leukocyte counts (PETO and PETO, 1972; COX, 1972).

A fuller description of these methods in non-mathematical language is given by PETO and PIKE (1972).

References

ADELSTEIN, A. M., DONOVAN, J. W.: Malignant disease in children whose mothers suffered chickenpox, mumps or rubella in pregnancy. Brit. med. J. **4**, 629 (1972).

BITHELL, J. F., DRAPER, G. J., GORBACH, P. D.: The association between malignant disease in children and maternal virus infections. Brit. med. J. **1**, 706 (1972).

COX, D. R.: Regression models and life tables. J. roy. statist. Soc. B **34**, 187 (1972).

FEDRICK, J., ALBERMAN, E. D.: Reported influenza in pregnancy and subsequent cancer in the child. Brit. med. J. **2**, 485 (1972).

MANTEL, N.: Evaluation of survival data and two new rank order statistics arising in its consideration. Cancer Chemother. Rep. **50**, 163 (1966).

Medical Research Council: Treatment of acute lymphoblastic leukaemia. Brit. med. J. **4**, 189 (1971).

Medical Research Council: 1st MRC myelomatosis trial. I. Analysis of presenting features of prognostic importance. Brit. J. Haemat. **24**, 123 (1972).

PETO, R., PETO, J.: Asymptotically efficient rank invariant test procedures. J. roy. statist. Soc. A **135**, 185 (1972).

PETO, R., PIKE, M. C.: Leukaemia trials. In: Medical surveys and clinical trials. 3rd Edition. Edited by S. C. TRUELOVE. To be published by Oxford University Press (1973).

STEWART, A., BARBER, R.: The epidemiological importance of childhood cancers. Brit. med. Bull. **27**, 64 (1971).

WALTERS, T. R., BUSHORE, M., SIMONE, J.: Poor prognosis in negro children with acute lymphocytic leukaemia. Cancer (Philad.) **29**, 210 (1972).

Third Session
Actuarial Results

Comparative Results Obtained in the Treatment of Acute Leukemia*

M. D. DOWLING, JR., M. HAGHBIN, T. S. GEE, B. CUNNINGHAM, C. T. C. TAN, B. D. CLARKSON, and J. H. BURCHENAL

Sloan-Kettering Institute for Cancer Research, Division of Chemotherapy Research, New York, NY/USA

The current programs used to treat acute leukemia at Memorial-Sloan Kettering Cancer Center are determined on the basis of morphologic criteria and age. The following report describes the regimens used and the current experience at this Center. Although age may be an important factor in the ultimate response of the patient, the morphologic characteristics of the disease govern the therapeutic approach. In acute lymphoblastic leukemia (ALL), the L-2 protocol is used. In the acute non-lymphoblastic leukemias, myeloblastic, myelomonoblastic and monoblastic (AML), the L-6 protocol is followed. The age division is based on practical lines in that there are both adult and pediatric leukemic groups. However, there are only minor differences in the protocols due mainly to practical rather than real considerations.

In lymphoblastic leukemia, it is now relatively easy to induce remissions. This is because leukemic lymphoblasts can generally be killed more or less selectively by certain drugs (e.g. prednisone, vincristine and L-asparaginase) while causing little damage to the normal hematopoietic precursors [4, 7, 12, 15]. With proper use of any of these three drugs the chemotherapist has the great advantage of being able to rapidly destroy a large fraction of leukemic lymphoblasts without causing serious and protracted injury to the normal marrow cells. Moreover, use of these drugs in combination or with other agents produces a higher remission rate than that achieved with one drug alone [4, 13, 15, 16].

In myeloblastic and related types of acute leukemia, these three drugs ordinarily have a negligible therapeutic effect, although occasional remissions may be obtained. Moreover, other non-cell cycle dependent agents also have relatively little selectivity of action for leukemic myeloblasts and may cause serious damage to the normal hematopoietic cells, which are generally already severely depleted by the disease [3, 9, 12, 15, 16]. The rate of movement of myeloblastic cells from the non-vulnerable G_1 state into S is so slow that it usually requires at least 6 to 8 days of treatment with

* This investigation was supported in part by USPHS Research Grants CA-05826 and CA-08748 from the National Cancer Institute, American Cancer Society Grant ET-2C, The John C. McCarroll Fund, Hearst Foundation Fund, and the United Leukemia Fund.

S-phase specific drugs to cause a remission and many normal precursors are killed in the process. Using either type of drug during attempted induction of remission gives the patient a high risk of dying from infection or hemorrhage due to depletion of granulocytes and platelets; drug-induced depression of the immune system may also contribute to greater susceptibility to infection.

One theoretical advantage of using S-phase specific drugs for remission induction in myeloblastic leukemia is that, during advanced disease, most of the normal hematopoietic stem cells are probably inhibited by the leukemic cells and are thus in an extended G_1 (or G_0) state and hence insensitive to such drugs [5,8], just like dormant leukemic cells. As many leukemic cells are killed, the normal stem cells are released from this inhibitory influence, reenter the cell cycle, and then become vulnerable. The second or third course of treatment with antimetabolites may cause significantly greater hematotoxicity than the first course (each course is generally separated by a treatment-free interval of about 2 weeks). It thus appears fairly certain that regenerating normal cells are often more vulnerable to these drugs, but there is little quantitative information yet available on the time relationships of their recovery after treatment with different drugs.

Thus in myeloblastic and related types of acute leukemia, because of the relative nonspecificity of the available drugs, the major unresolved problem is how to kill enough leukemic cells to cause a remission without at the same time producing intolerable damage to the normal hematopoietic and immune systems. Good supportive care, platelet and granulocyte transfusions, antibiotics, and possibly a protected environment are important adjuncts, but even under the most favorable circumstances the risk of death is high during attempted induction of remission.

Once remission has been achieved in either type of acute leukemia, the objective becomes the elimination of all the surviving leukemic cells; although a billion or more may remain, only the stem cells have unlimited proliferative capability and attention must be focused on these.

There are three main obstacles to the goal of eliminating all the leukemic cells:

1. Drug resistance may develop, so that some leukemic cells survive exposure to drug concentrations which were initially cytocidal to most of them. To try to prevent development of resistance to any one drug, it would seem logical to use combinations of drugs concurrently, or else sequential courses of treatment with different drugs having different mechanisms of action.

2. In some patients, leukemic cells may become sequestered in sanctuaries, especially the central nervous system, into which most drugs fail to penetrate in effective lethal concentrations. Previous attempts at treating symptomatic (i.e. advanced) central nervous system disease have oenerally had only limited and temporary success. Therefore several current regimens include prophylactic intrathecal chemotherapy (and/or x-irradiation to the neuroaxis) during the initial course of remission induction, before leukemic infiltration of the central nervous system has become well established [1, 2, 17]. It is as yet uncertain how vigorous or protracted such therapy must be in order to permanently sterilize the central nervous system of leukemic cells.

3. The third major obstacle is the persistence of a small but significant fraction of leukemic cells in an extended G_1 phase, in which state they are relatively insensitive to the cytotoxic agents. No reliable way has yet been found to eliminate these long-term dormant cells.

Since no better way has yet been found to eliminate the resting leukemic cells, probably the best therapeutic strategies at present are: [1] to reduce the leukemic population as much as possible by "consolidating" the remission during the initial treatment regimen; [2] to incorporate in the maintenance regimen periodic administration of a non-cell cycle dependent agent in as high dosage as tolerable, since such agents are at least partially effective in killing resting cells; and [3] to continue fairly intensive chemotherapy for several years after good remission has been induced, using different drugs in rotation in as high dosage as tolerated to reduce the likelihood of development of drug resistance. It is probably best to use short (4 or 5 day) courses of treatment interrupted by treatment-free intervals to allow recovery of normal hematopoietic cells; the periods without treatment should be kept as short as possible to minimize regrowth of leukemic cells. The hope of such continuing treatment is that all of the resting leukemic cells will eventually reenter a sensitive phase of the cell cycle at a time coinciding with the achievement of a high concentration of a drug whose cytocidal effect is maximal during that portion of the cycle.

The L-2 Protocol

The current treatment (L-2) protocol we are using at Memorial Hospital for lymphoblastic leukemia is shown in Figs. 1 and 2. The initial results are encouraging [11], but we have only been using this regimen for a little over 2 years and cannot predict the long-term results. Undoubtedly, improvements can be made, and we plan to modify the protocol as its weaknesses become apparent.

The protocol was designed for patients who have had no previous treatment, and it is assumed that in all such patients the leukemic cells will have some sensitivity to each component of the regimen (except possibly L-asparaginase). Short of interrupting the protocol after each phase of treatment and following the marrow serially to estimate the rate of relapse, there is no technique to evaluate the effectiveness of each component of the regimen separately.

INTENSIVE "L-2" TREATMENT PROTOCOL FOR ACUTE LYMPHOBLASTIC LEUKEMIA

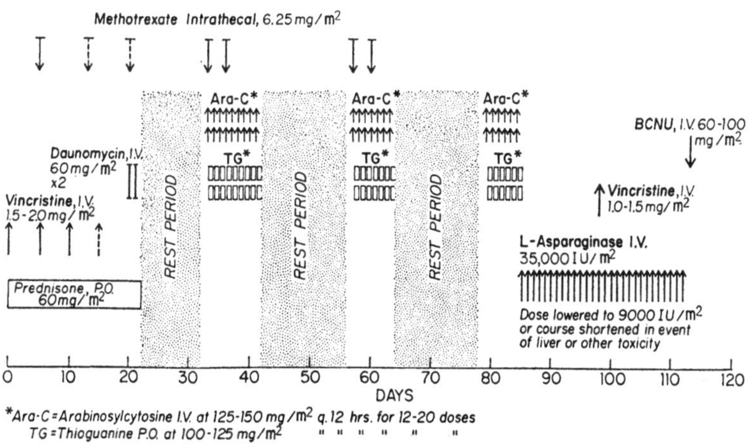

Fig. 1. The L-2 Protocol (Part I)

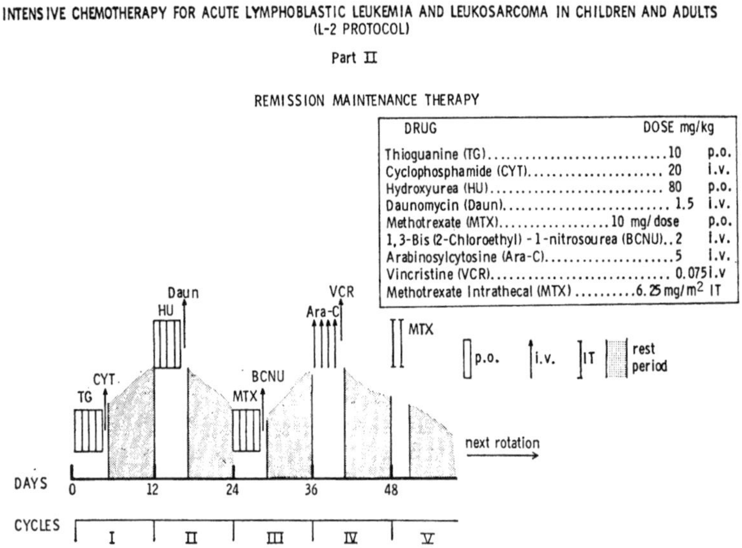

Fig. 2. The L-2 Protocol (Part II)

The initial treatment is prednisone and vincristine, since these drugs in combination are known to produce remissions in approximately 85% of untreated patients and to cause less damage to the normal cells than most other agents [13, 15]. In a few patients the marrow will not yet be in complete remission, but almost all (previously untreated) patients have at least a partial response and are better able to tolerate subsequent therapy with more toxic drugs. Two large doses of Daunomycin are then given (while continuing prednisone). After the patient has recovered from Daunomycin toxicity, therapy is then started with a combination of arabinosyl cytosine and thioguanine [10], giving both drugs every 12 hours to prevent any leukemic cells from completing DNA synthesis between attainment of cytocidal blood concentrations. Although there is considerable variation among patients in the duration of therapy needed to cause marrow depression, most cannot safely tolerate more than about 7 to 10 days of such treatment (14 to 20 doses). Repeated courses of arabinosyl cytosine and thioguanine are given in order to kill as many of the actively dividing leukemic cells as possible. A 1 to 3 week period of rest is necessary between each course of treatment to allow the normal marrow cells to recover. L-Asparaginase is started immediately after the third course of arabinosyl cytosine and thioguanine. Although the optimal therapeutic dose is not yet known [7], we have chosen to use moderately high doses until more information is available on this point. L-Asparaginase is continued for 28 days in the hope that the majority of leukemic cells will begin proliferating during this period and be destroyed. One disadvantage of such a long course of treatment is, of course, that in some patients the leukemic cells will not be sensitive to this agent and that in such cases there may occur significant regrowth of the leukemic population; it is therefore probably advisable to administer one or more doses of another cytotoxic drug (e.g. vincristine) concurrently with L-asparaginase to prevent such an occurrence.

To try to eliminate the (presumed) remaining leukemic cells after completing Part I of the protocol, patients are then started on Part II as outlined in Fig. 2. In this sense, "maintenance therapy" is a misnomer, since the main objective of this continuing therapy is to eradicate all of the residual leukemic cells. Since it is not know how long leukemic cells may remain resting and hence survive, our present plan calls for continuing this treatment for at least 3 years.

In view of the complexity of the L-2 protocol and the high drug doses employed, it is perhaps surprising that it is generally well tolerated and that severe toxicity has been rare [11]. On the other hand, it should be emphasized that it is not a protocol that can be followed by rote, as there is considerable variation among patients in the amount of therapy that can be tolerated. While the general outline shown in Figs. 1 and 2 is adhered to as closely as possible, it is often necessary to modify the treatment in accordance with the patient's hematologic condition. Blood counts and marrows must be followed closely, and the treatment schedule is in effect individualized; in many patients it is necessary to lower the drug dosage or delay starting the next cycle of treatment until the hematologic status has improved. Although no patients with lymphoblastic leukemia have died from drug toxicity on the L-2 protocol, we have had at least one death from drug toxicity when using the L-6 protocol during the remission consolidation phase in a patient with myeloblastic leukemia. Thus, the hazard of this or similar intensive treatment regimens is real, and we agree with Holland that such therapy should be carried out in specialized treatment centers under the close supervision of highly experienced personnel [14].

Results with the L-2 Protocol

The protocol was initiated in November, 1969 and 46 untreated children (< 15 years old) have been adequately treated. At this time, 2 are too early to evaluate. Of the remaining 44 all achieved an M_1 marrow and all but 1 a complete remission.

DURATION OF REMISSION WITH L-2 PROTOCOL

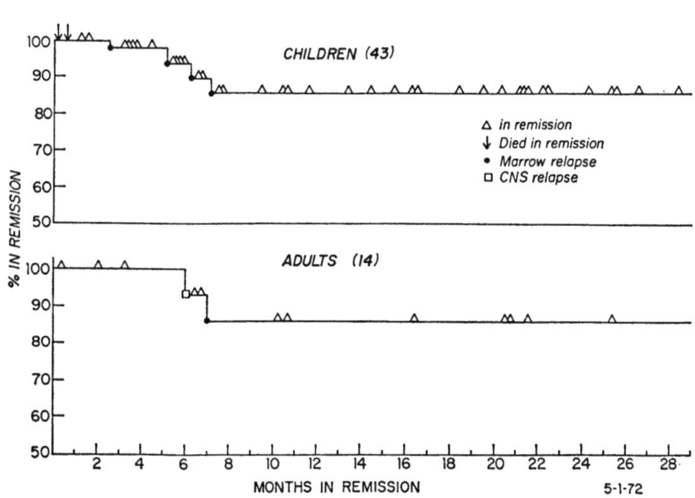

Fig. 3

Remissions are continuing from 1 to 29 months. Two children died in remission of serum hepatitis and 4 patients relapsed, 2 of whom died failing other therapy.

There are 38 patients who are free of disease, including the central nervous system, for 29 months. Fourteen are greater than 1 year and 5 greater than 2 years (Fig. 3).

There have been 17 previously untreated or minimally pretreated adults. Fourteen achieved remissions and 12 are continuing in remission at 1 to 24 months. There have been 2 deaths in persons age 63 and 78 who were inadequately treated. One 16-year-old youth failed the protocol. One patient in remission developed meningeal leukemia at 7 month and 1 had systemic relapse at 8 months (Fig. 3).

Thirty-eight children and adults who had been previously treated were entered into this study. The rate and duration of response were not favorable as compared to the previously untreated or minimally pretreated patients. There were 18 complete remissions and 7 good partial remissions. These patients have been in remission from 1 to 30 months. There have been 11 relapses varying in time from 7 days to 30 months.

Central Nervous System Prophylaxis

In awareness that most drugs used systematically fail to reach the meninges in effective cytocidal concentrations, prophylactic intrathecal therapy has been used. The first dose of intrathecal methotrexate 6.25 mg/m² is administered on the 4th day of induction (Fig. 1). Two to 3 more doses are given during the vincristine–prednisone

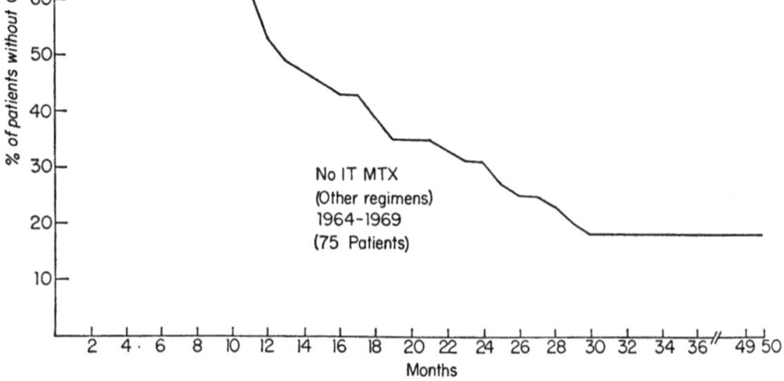

Fig. 4. Incidence of Central Nervous System Disease With L-2 and Other Regimens in Acute Lymphoblastic Leukemia in Children

induction usually 2 to 3 days apart. Further intrathecal methotrexate is given during the initial two courses of arabinosyl cytosine and thioguanine for a grand total of 7 to 8 planned doses. No serious side effects have been observed. The main reactions have been headache, backache and vomiting. Only one convulsive episode occurred and it could not be clearly attributed to intrathecal methotrexate. The same child has remained asymptomatic with subsequent instillations. It should be noted that, in the pediatric group, further intrathecal methotrexate is given with each rotation of part II of the protocol. However, the adult patients receive no further intrathecal injections once part I of the protocol is completed.

Although it is still much too early to be sure of this mode of CNS prophylaxis, a comparison with our previous experience of the development of meningeal leukemia (Fig. 4) speaks favorably for this form of prophylaxis combined with the L-2 protocol.

The L-6 Protocol

Beginning in May, 1970, all new adults with AML seen at Memorial Hospital were entered on the "L-6" protocol consisting of repeated courses of arabinosyl cytosine 3 mg/kg by intravenous injection, plus thioguanine 2.5 mg/kg orally, each given every 12 hours until induction of remission. Once an M_1 marrow is achieved, three subsequent courses of arabinosyl cytosine and thioguanine are given, each to moderate hypocellularity of the marrow as consolidation. The L-6 maintenance follows with a complex rotation sequence of multiple drugs: vincristine, methotrexate, 1-3 bis (2-chloro-ethyl)-1-nitrosourea, hydroxyurea, Daunomycin, arabinosyl cytosine and thioguanine (Fig. 5).

INTENSIVE "L-6" TREATMENT PROTOCOL FOR ACUTE MYELOBLASTIC LEUKEMIA
(Revised 1972)

INDUCTION + CONSOLIDATION

Drug	Dose
Arabinosylcytosine (Ara-C)	3.0mg/kg q 12hr. i.v.
Thioguanine (TG)	2.5mg/kg q 12hr. p.o.

MAINTENANCE

Drug	Dose
Vincristine (VCR)	0.03-0.04 mg/kg i.v.
Methotrexate (MTX)	10 mgx4 p.o.
BCNU (1,3-Bis(2-chloroethyl)-1-nitrosourea	1.0-2.0 mg/kg i.v.
Thioguanine (TG)	10 mg/kgx4 p.o.
Cytoxan (CTX)	10-20 mg/kg i.v.
Hydroxyurea (HU)	60-80 mg/kgx4 p.o.
Daunorubicin (Daun)	1.0 mg/kg i.v.

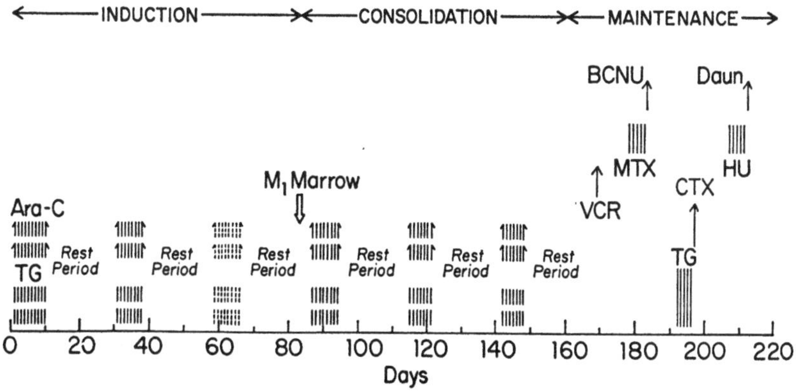

Fig. 5. The L-6 Protocol

The rationales for designing and implementing the L-6 protocol were as follows:

1. Selective Anti-leukemic Activity of Arabinosyl cytosine and Thioguanine: The efficacy of arabinosyl cytosine and thioguanine for inducing remissions is more consistent than any other regimen we had tried; for reasons as yet unknown, it appears that this combination of antimetabolites causes more selective damage to (AML) leukemic cells than any single agent or other combination of agents.

2. Duration of S-Phase and Spacing of Drug Doses: The duration of the DNA synthetic period (S-phase) of acute leukemic cells is about 20 hours, at least during advanced disease [6]. Since both arabinosyl cytosine and thioguanine are probably lethal only to cells in S, the drug doses were therefore spaced 12 hours apart to prevent any cells from completing S without being exposed to (presumed) cytocidal drug concentration.

3. Doses of Arabinosyl cytosine and Thioguanine: The same doses used in the once-daily arabinosyl cytosine and thioguanine series were given every 12 hours, since it was already evident from this original trial that these doses were cytocidal for most human leukemic cells. An additional reason for using "full" doses twice dailey was that in the initial series we had encountered some patients whose disease was primarily resistant to once-daily arabinosyl cytosine and thioguanine, and it was thereby hoped that primary drug resistance would be avoided. If the drug concentrations are sufficiently high to be lethal to all cells entering S, there should be no sublethally affected surviving cells and less likelihood for emergence of a resistant population. It might be argued that even higher doses ought to be still more effective, but prior experience with most cytotoxic drugs has shown that any selective anti-leukemic effect is usually lost with very high doses. More extensive comparative trials will, of course, be necessary to establish the optimal drug doses which may vary in individual patients.

4. Duration of First Course of Arabinosyl cytosine and Thioguanine: Whenever possible, the first course of arabinosyl cytosine and thioguanine was continued until it was estimated that at least 90% of the leukemic population had been destroyed and that the marrow would become moderately to severely hypocellular. Since experience showed that maximum marrow depression generally occurred about 10 to 14 days after interrupting treatment, the decision when to stop was partly expectant. Experience has shown that the first sign of less than normal marrow cellularity is the stop signal. As in the original series of patients treated with (once-daily) arabinosyl cytosine and thioguanine, the duration of the first course of treatment was individualized and depended on the patient's general condition, hematologic status and rapidity of therapeutic response; most patients received between 15 and 35 doses. Sometimes, if serious infectious or bleeding complications developed, treatment was temporarily interrupted before the desired degree of leukemic cell kill was reached. When it was estimated that close to maximum tolerated therapy had been given, a rest period averaging 2 to 3 weeks was then allowed to permit regeneration of the normal hematopoietic cells.

The situation is often precarious during the first course of treatment, because there are usually few normal precursors remaining in the marrow at the time of diagnosis and most of these are killed by the treatment. The patient thus has a high risk of dying as a result of further depletion of granulocytes and platelets. Vigorous supportive therapy is essential during this critical period, but once there has been an opportunity for regeneration of adequate numbers of granulocytes and platelets, the partial remission can then be consolidated relatively safely.

5. Subsequent Courses of Arabinosyl cytosine and Thioguanine: Repeated courses of arabinosyl cytosine and thioguanine are given to destroy as many leukemic cells as possible. A rest period of about 2 to 3 weeks must be allowed in between each course of arabinosyl cytosine and thioguanine to allow regeneration of the normal cells. These rest periods allow the (previously dormant) leukemic cells that escaped being killed by the first course to resume proliferating and become vulnerable to the drugs [6]. Although there is little quantitative or temporal information available, it is probable that, after the marrow has been depleted by the first course of therapy, both the surviving leukemic cells and the normal stem cells begin proliferating at faster rates than prior to treatment [6]. Thus both populations should be more vulnerable to subsequent treatment with arabinosyl cytosine and thioguanine. Because the normal cells may be more vulnerable, subsequent courses of treatment must be given cautiously; generally no more than 12 to 20 doses are safely tolerated, even if the granulocyte and platelet counts are normal or supranormal (i.e. due to rebound) when treatment is resumed. We often stop subsequent courses when the granulocyte and/or platelet counts and marrow are near normal or only moderately depressed, knowing that the nadir of depression will usually occur about 10 to 14 days later. A rest period of several weeks is then permitted, and after the marrow and peripheral blood counts have again recovered, the process is repeated until the marrow is in a good (M_1) remission.

6. Multiple Sequential Drug Maintenance Regimen: Because of the problems inherent in the prolonged use of arabinosyl cytosine and thioguanine, we have designed a regimen employing a complex sequence of other cytotoxic drugs which can be carried out on an outpatient basis (Fig. 5). Each drug is given in the sequence shown in as high a dosage as can be safely tolerated, and the sequence is continued in rotation indefinitely. In general, the therapeutic tactics in this part of the protocol are to administer a 4-day course of a cell cycle-specific agent in as high dosage as tolerated to kill any leukemic cells which have resumed dividing. On the fifth day, a single dose of a cycle nonspecific agent is then given to try to destroy residual dormant cells. It would be preferable to continue the cycle-specific agent for longer than 4 days, but this is usually not possible because of toxicity at the high doses used. Relatively high doses are given to try to avoid early development of drug resistance and different drugs are used in rotation for the same reason. There may be some cross-resistance between some of the agents, and we are also limited here by the availability of only a few oral cycle-specific drugs effective in AML.

The first patients treated with the L-6 protocol were given only one additional course of arabinosyl cytosine and thioguanine after induction of an (M_1) marrow remission. They were then discharged and given one (incomplete) sequence of therapy with the maintenance regimen as outpatients and then readmitted for another course of arabinosyl cytosine and thioguanine followed immediately by L-asparaginase. However, as we gained experience with the L-6 protocol, it became apparent that the multiple additional drug sequence was effective in maintaining remissions *only* if the remission was already well established. We are therefore now routinely giving 3 courses of arabinosyl cytosine and thioguanine *after* achievement of an M_1 marrow remission prior to beginning the maintenance regimen. We have also now excluded

L-asparaginase entirely because it lacks significant therapeutic activity in AML and may cause liver and other toxicity. Thus, after recovery from the third "consolidation" (post M_1 marrow) course or arabinosyl cytosine and thioguanine, patients are now placed immediately on the maintenance regimen, beginning with vincristine and continuing the sequence in rotation indefinitely.

Results with the L-6 Protocol

As of June 1, 1972, 43 previously untreated patients with AML have been entered on the L-6 protocol. The median and mean ages were respectively 46 and 41 years (range 16 to 67). Forty-two trials have been completed; 1 patient has just recently started. Of the 42 completed trials, 28 patients have had remissions (25 complete and 3 good partial), 10 died during attempted induction, and 5 failed. In 2, the trial was clearly a failure since the marrow was still not in remission after 5 adequate courses of arabinosyl cytosine and thioguanine. One withdrew after a failure following one course, and 2 others failed after 3 courses and were induced with other chemotherapeutic agents.

In the 28 patients having remissions, M_1 marrow status was achieved after a mean of 2 courses (range 1 to 5) and a mean of 35 doses (range 15 to 105). Two patients died while in remission: one, a 35-year-old woman, died of a fulminating pneumonia at the end of the first consolidation course of arabinosyl cytosine and thioguanine (after achievement of an M_1 marrow), just after completing L-asparaginase. The other, a 62-year-old priest with known severe arteriosclerotic heart disease, died from complications resulting from an unrelated cardiovascular accident while in remission. Of the remaining 26 patients achieving remission, the marrow has just recently reached an M_1 status in 1 patient, and the others are continuing in remission for 2 to 23 months as of June 1, 1972, five of them for over 12 months (Fig. 6).

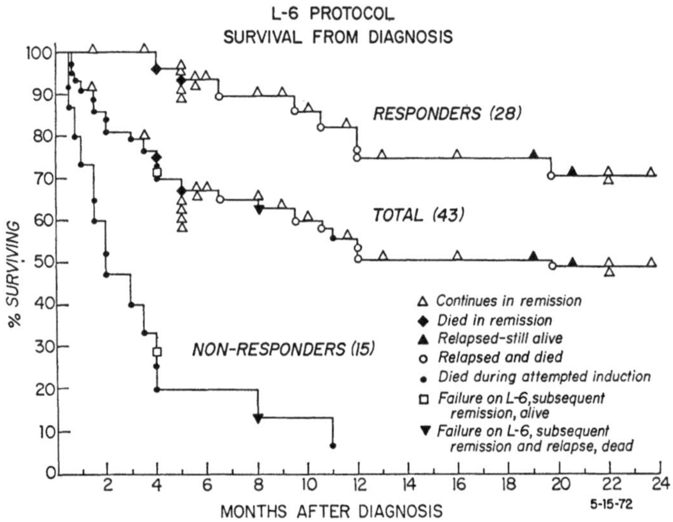

Fig. 6. Survival From Diagnosis With the L-6 Protocol

In 8 patients the disease has relapsed. Two had a total of only 2 courses of arabinosyl cytosine and thioguanine and relapse occurred while they were receiving interim maintenance therapy. In retrospect, it appears obvious that the arabinosyl cytosine and thioguanine therapy was inadequate and that in neither patient was the marrow in a good remission prior to their starting the maintenance regimen. It had been planned to readmit both patients for one or more additional courses of arabinosyl cytosine and thioguanine but this was delayed because the first patient returned temporarily to her home in Peru an the second developed serum hepatitis.

It was our unfortunate experience with these two patients that prompted us to alter the protocol, and all patients are now receiving 3 courses of arabinosyl cytosine and thioguanine after attainment of an M_1 marrow prior to beginning maintenance therapy.

Of the other 6 relapsed patients, 4 completed the entire L-6 protocol. One who had been in remission 18 months at the time of relapse has subsequently been reinduced with the L-6 protocol and is receiving consolidation therapy at this time. Two others in remission for 17 and 14 months never received L-asparaginase as part of their initial program: one refused because of fear of side effects and the other developed seum hepatitis just prior to therapy. The former relapsed and died of a cerebral hemorrhage and the latter has achieved an M_2 marrow with a reinduction attempt with the L-6 protocol and is still receiving therapy.

The results with twice daily arabinosyl cytosine and thioguanine have been much less satisfactory in previously treated patients. Forty eight trials have been started in 42 patients. Nineteen had remission; 7 relapsed in several months (all had previously had arabinosyl cytosine and thioguanine), 1 died in remission (of fungal brain abscesses), and 11 are still in remission after 1 to 12 months. There were 29 failures. These 29 non-responders included fifteen patients who had had greater than 6 months of pretreatment with arabinosyl cytosine and thioguanine. A sixteenth patient had previously been treated with 6-mercaptopurine. Eighteen of the 29 non-responders died during attempted induction with arabinosyl cytosine and thioguanine, 1 subsequently had a 5-month remission on other chemotherapy, and 2 are presently receiving other chemotherapy. The remaining 8 died while receiving different chemotherapy.

From our experience thus far, it appears that the disease definitely may become refractóry to arabinosyl cytosine and thioguanine every 12 hours in patients who have previously been adequately treated with these drugs, and that the best chance of success is in patients who have not had prior exposure to either drug.

The results so far in previously untreated patients are superior to those in other regimens we have tried including arabinosyl cytosine and thioguanine once daily. The remission induction period is frequently very hazardous; about 60% of the patients who eventually had good remissions developed serious infections or other complications during this period and survived these crises only with the aid of vigorous and meticulous supportive therapy. The dosage schedule of arabinosyl cytosine and thioguanine is very toxic to normal marrow cells, and the regimen is far from ideal for remission induction. However, until a less toxic regimen with equal or greater therapeutic effectiveness is discovered, this one appears to be as good as or better than any other in AML.

The quality (i.e. completeness in terms of reduction of leukemic population) and duration of remission are as important as the frequency of occurrence, and while we are optimistic, it is too soon to know how long the present remissions will last. We are convinced that intensive treatment following achievement of an M_1 marrow offers the best chance for a longlasting remission, but we are still uncertain as to the best means to accomplish this and plan to continue trying different therapeutic strategies.

References

1. AUR, R., HUSTU, O., VERZOSA, M., SIMONE, J.: A comparative study of "prophylactic" craniospinal irradiation in 94 children with acute lymphocytic leukemia. Proc. Amer. Ass. Cancer Res. **12**, 19 (1971).
2. AUR, R. J. A., SIMONE, J., HUSTU, H. O., WALTERS, T., BURELLA, L., PRATT, C., PINDEL, D.: Central nervous system therapy and combination chemotherapy of childhood lymphocytic leukemia. Blood (in press).
3. BERNARD, J., JACQUILLART, C., WEIL, M., BOIRON, M., TANZER, J.: Present results on donaurubicin (rubidomycin, Donaumycin). Recent Results in Cancer Research. Advances in the treatment of acute (Blastic) leukemias, p. 3. Ed.: G. MATHÉ. New York: Springer 1970.
4. BURCHENAL, J. H.: Clinical evaluation and future prospects of asparaginase. Recent Results in Cancer Research. Advances in the treatment of acute (Blastic) leukemias, p. 20. Ed.: G. MATHÉ. New York: Springer 1970.
5. CLARKSON, B. D., FRIED, J., STRIFE, A., SAKAI, Y., OTA, K., OHKITA, T., MASUDA, R.: Studies of cellular proliferation in human leukemia. IV. Behavior of normal hematopoietic cells in three adults with acute leukemia given continuous infusions of ^{3}H-thymidine. Cancer (Philad.) **26**, 1 (1970) .
6. CLARKSON, B. D., FRIED, J.: Changing concepts of treatment in acute leukemia. Medical Clinics of North America, vol. 55, p. 561. Philadelphia-London-Toronto: W. B. Saunders Company 1971.
7. CLARKSON, B., KRAKOFF, I., BURCHENAL, J., KARNOFSKY, D., GOLBEY, R., OETTGEN, H., DOWLING, M., LIPTON, A.: Clinical results of treatment with E. Coli L-asparaginase in adults with leukemia, lymphoma, and solid tumors. Cancer (Philad.) **25**, 279 (1970).
8. CLARKSON, B. D., OHKITA, T., OTA, K., FRIED, J.: Studies of cellular proliferation in human leukemia. I. Estimation of growth rates of leukemic and normal hematopoietic cells in two adults with acute leukemia given single injections of tritiated thymidine. J. clin. Invest. **46**, 506 (1967).
9. FREIREICH, E. J., BODEY, G. P., HART, J. S., RODRIGUEZ, V., WHITECAR, J. P., FREI, E. III.: Remission induction in adults with acute myelogenous leukemia. Recent Results in Cancer Research. Advances in the treatment of acute (Blastic) leukemias, p. 85. Ed.: G. MATHÉ. New York: Springer 1970.
10. GEE, T. S., YU, K.-P., CLARKSON, B. D.: Treatment of adult acute leukemia with arabinosyl cytosine and thioguanine. Cancer (Philad.) **23**, 1019 (1969).
11. HAGHBIN, M., TAN, C., GEE, T., DOWLING, M., CLARKSON, B., SIDHU, J., MURPHY, M. L., BURCHENAL, J., SYKES, M.: Sequential intensive drug therapy in acute lymphoblastic leukemia (ALL) and leukosarcoma (LSA). Proc. Amer. Ass. Cancer Res. **12**, 122 (1971).
12. HENDERSON, E. S.: Treatment of acute leukemia. Sem. Hemat. **6**, 271 (1969).
13. HENDERSON, E. S., SAMAHA, R. J.: Evidence that drugs in multiple combinations have materially advanced the treatment of human malignancies. Cancer Res. **29**, 2272 (1969).
14. HOLLAND, J. F.: Who should treat acute leukemia? J. Amer. med. Ass. **209**, 1511 (1969).
15. HOLLAND, J. F., GLIDEWELL, O.: Complementary chemotherapy in acute leukemia. Recent Results in Cancer Research. Advances in the treatment of acute (Blastic) leukemias, p. 95. Ed.: G. MATHÉ. New York: Springer 1970.
16. Leukemia and Hematosarcoma Cooperative Group of the European Organisation for Research on the Treatment of Cancer (E. O. R. T. C.): Rubidomycin (or daunomycin): A clinical evaluation. Recent Results in Cancer Research. Advances in the treatment of acute (Blastic) leukemias, p. 9. Ed.: G. MATHÉ. New York: Springer 1970.
17. MATHÉ, G., AMIEL, J. L., SCHWARZENBERG, L., SCHNEIDER, M., CATTAN, A., HAYAT, M., DE VASSAL, F., SCHLUMBERGER, J. R.: Methods and strategy for the treatment of acute lymphoblastic leukemia. Recent Results in Cancer Research. Advances in the treatment of acute (Blastic) leukemias, p. 109. Ed.: G. MATHÉ. New York: Springer 1970.

Clinical and Immunological Recovery of Children with Acute Lymphocytic Leukemia Admitted to "Total Therapy" Studies*

L. Borella, A. A. Green, R. J. A. Aur, J. V. Simone, and D. Pinkel

St. Jude Children's Research Hospital, Memphis, TN/USA

"Total Therapy" studies of childhood leukemia were initiated in 1962 at St. Jude Children's Research Hospital, Memphis, Tenn., USA, with the immediate goals of increasing remission rate, prolonging duration of complete remission, and achieving a significant rate of permanent cure.

The principal features of these studies have included administration of combination chemotherapy and "prophylactic" central nervous system (CNS) irradiation and the use of biological parameters for determining drug dosage in individual patients. Over 350 children have entered this program in the past 10 years.

The purpose of this paper is to present the long-term results of our 1962—1970 studies and to answer the following questions:

1. What is the earliest and most accurate indicator of long-term *leukemia-free* survival?

2. What are the prospects for permanent complete remission after stopping chemotherapy?

3. Do patients become fully immunocompetent when chemotherapy is discontinued after 3 years? What cellular immunological events occur during and after cessation of treatment? Is there any correlation between immunological recovery and duration of remission?

Descriptions of our patients, our criteria for diagnosis and remission, and methods of "total therapy" studies have been reported previously in detail [1—9]. The general procedure consisted of:

1. Induction of complete remission, usually with prednisone and vincristine. The remission rates ranged from 87 to 92%.

2. Multiple-agent combination chemotherapy with MP, MTX and cyclo for 2 to 3 years.

3. "Prophylatic" CNS irradiation early during remission. Doses of 500 to 1200 rads did not prevent CNS leukemia, but a 2400 rads dose was proven to be effective.

---

* Supported by Grants CA-05176, CA-08480 and CA-12787-01, CA-08151 from the National Cancer Institute, and by ALSAC.

We defined *complete remission duration* as the time from initial complete remission to the first sign of relapse, whether hematologic, *CNS* or visceral. Hematologic remission duration is the time from first complete remission bone marrow to first evidence of hematologic relapse. This may include periods of CNS or visceral relapse. Survival time is the period from diagnosis to death.

A. Long-Term Leukemia-Free Survival

Of 41 patients who entered studies I—III (1962—1965) and 37 who attained remission, 7 have been in continuous complete remission for 7 to 9 years. Do these 7 children simply represent the far end of an exponential slope that steadily decreases until no children remain in remission or survive? To examine this question, the log of the percentage of patients remaining in complete remission, in hematologic remission and surviving was plotted against time. As shown in Fig. 1, the slopes differ in the rate of descent, but each virtually describes a straight line to about 20%. After 28 months the percentage of patients in complete remission has remained constant with no additional relapses. The hematologic remission and survival slopes descend more slowly, but steadily approach and meet the horizontal complete remission slope years later. This is evidence for what one might logically expect: *complete remission duration is the earliest and most accurate clinical parameter for predicting long-term leukemia-free survival.* After $2^1/_2$ years in these studies, one-half of the patients were alive and one-third were still in hematologic remission. But only 7 were in continuous

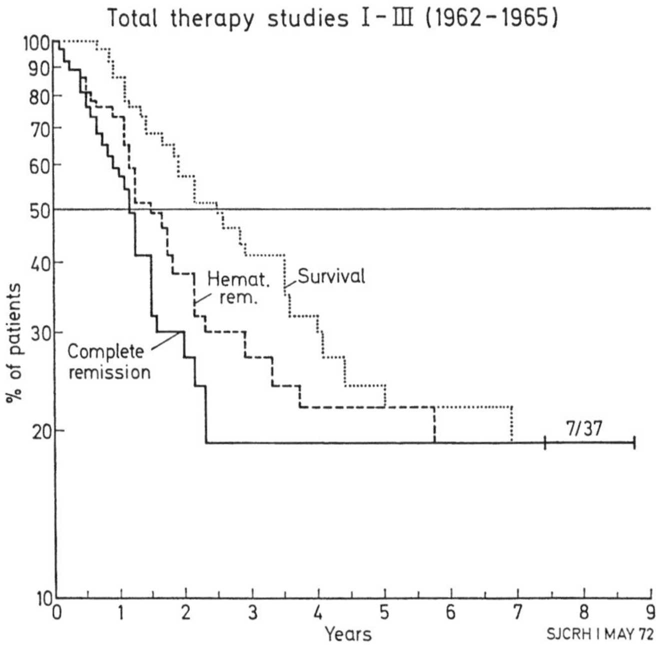

Fig. 1. Total therapy studies I—III (1962—1965). Cross marks (1) indicate range of complete remission duration. See text for definitions

complete remission and all 7 have remained in remission for an additional 5 to 7 years after cessation of therapy.

What rate of leukemia-free survival can be expected for patients who received effective "prophylactic" CNS therapy? Fig. 2 is a semi-log plot of complete remission duration for patients in studies I—III who received inadequate CNS irradiation, patients in V and VI who received 2400 rads of CNS irradiation and the control patients in study VI who did not receive irradiation. Despite the fact that studies I—III and study VI-not irradiated were initiated 6 years apart, the complete remis-

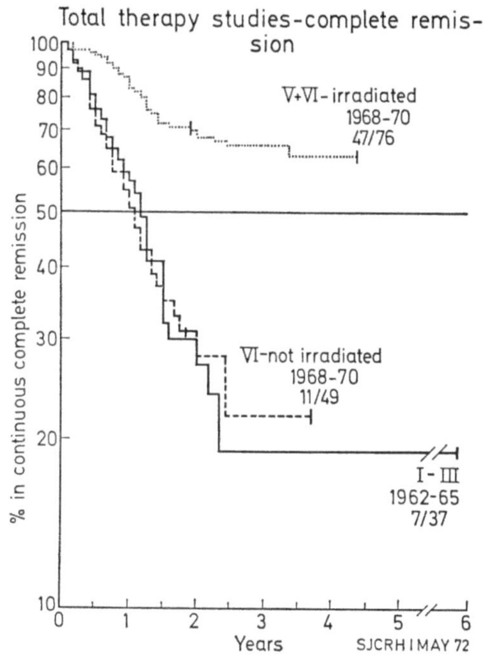

Fig. 2. Total therapy studies — complete remission. Cross marks (1) indicate range of complete remission duration. See text for definition of complete remission

sion slopes are virtually identical from the first months on, apparently not affected by more recent modifications of chemotherapy such as periodic "reinduction pulses" and supportive care such as newer antibiotics. Patients in studies V and VI-irradiated describe a strikingly different slope. Over 60% of these patients have been in complete remission for 2 to 4 years. Even more important, however, the slope appears to be leveling off. If the trend continues, it is reasonable to expect that 50% of these patients will enjoy long-term leukemia-free survival.

B. Relapses Following Cessation of Therapy

It has been the policy at this institution to discontinue chemotherapy after 2 to 3 years of continuous complete remission. Treatment has been stopped in 35 patients from studies I to V (1962—1968). In addition, chemotherapy was discontinued in another seven children who were treated according to study V (1967—1968) but who were not included in that study because they had received other forms of chemotherapy before admission. Thus, we have evaluated the duration of remission in 42 children with ALL whose chemotherapy was terminated after 2 to 3 years of CCR (Table 1). The first group of patients had received "prophylactic" CNS irradiation in doses ranging from 500 to 2400 rads (studies I, II, III and V). A second group did not receive "prophylactic" irradiation and the third group was treated according to the study V protocol, but had received prior chemotherapy.

Table 1. Cessation of therapy after 2 to 3 years of continuous complete remission in 42 children with ALL (studies I to V)

	"Prophylactic" CNS radiation	No previous therapy	Number patients	Duration of continuous complete remission (years)	Time of theraphy (years)	Relapses no.	%
First group	+	+	27	$\underline{4^2/_{12}}$ ($3^{10}/_{12}$—$8^6/_{12}$)	$\underline{1^6/_{12}}$ ($^8/_{12}$—$5^6/_{12}$)	2	7
Second group	−	+	8	$\underline{3^4/_{12}}$ ($3^2/_{12}$—6)	$\underline{^9/_{12}}$ ($^2/_{12}$—3)	6	75
Third group	+	−	7	$\underline{4}$ ($3^6/_{12}$—$4^4/_{12}$)	$\underline{1}$ ($^7/_{12}$—$1^4/_{12}$)	1	14

"Prophylactic" CNS radiation was given early in remission in doses ranging from 500 rads (Studies I and II) to 2400 rads (Study V). The third group received other forms of chemotherapy before receiving the Total Therapy V Regimen. Median is underlined. Range is in parenthesis.

Of the 27 children treated from the beginning with combination chemotherapy and CNS irradiation, only two relapses (7%) occurred after the drugs were stopped. The rest remain in continuous complete remission for periods ranging from $3^1/_2$ to $8^1/_2$ years. In contrast, of the eight patients who had not received "prophylactic" irradiation, six relapsed after the treatment was discontinued. Although the numbers are small, these results suggest that patients who do not receive "prophylactic" CNS irradiation are at high risk for relapse after therapy is stopped. On the other hand, patients who receive CNS irridiation early during remission have a lower risk of relapse subsequent to cessation of treatment.

C. Immunological Rebound Following Cessation of Therapy

In vivo and *in vitro* studies were performed in patients "on" and "off" therapy with the aim of elucidating the immunological events that occur when chemotherapy is stopped after 2 to 3 years of immunosuppression [7—9]. We also asked whether or not there was a relationship between recovery of immunocompetence and prolonged leukemia-free survival. A summary of these studies [8, 9] is presented in Table 2.

Table 2. Immunological rebound following cessation of 2½ to 3 years of theraphy [8, 9, 10]

A. In vivo

1. Early increase of bone marrow (BM) lymphocytes followed by slow rise of peripheral blood (PB) lymphocytes
2. Rise of IgM and IgG serum levels within 2 to 4 months
3. Antibody production without extrinsic antigenic stimulation

B. In vitro response by marrow and blood lymphocytes

1. Increase in % of responders, but not in magnitude of response, to phytohemagglutinin
2. Increase in both % of responders and magnitude of response to the antigens (Keyhole Limpet Hemocyanin, Candida, Flu virus)
3. Phytohemagglutinin-responsive cells and antigen-responsive cells have different kinetics of recovery and are differently distributed in bone marrow and peripheral blood.

After cessation of therapy, we observed an immunological rebound with the following characteristics:

1. There was an early increase of bone marrow lymphocytes (higher than 40% in some patients) followed by a slow rise of peripheral *blood lymphocytes.* This suggests that repopulation of *immunocompetent* cells originates in the bone marrow compartment.

2. IgM and IgG serum immunoglobulins increased following cessation of treatment. At the same time there was a rise of antibody titer to influenza virus, an antigen to which these children were exposed more than 1 year earlier.

3. There was a rebound of cell-mediated immunity as assayed by the response of peripheral blood and bone marrow lymphocytes to blastogenic stimulation with PHA and various antigens.

4. No differences were found between the characteristics of the immunological rebound after cessation of chemotherapy in three children who subsequently relapsed and those who had remained in complete remission.

From these observations, we have drawn several implications. An increase of bone marrow lymphocytes above 40% in children with ALL in whom chemotherapy has been discontinued does not indicate relapse but is probably a manifestation of immunological recovery. When drugs are stopped because of infection, a rise in antibody titers possibly reflects immune rebound to an "old" antigen and is not necessarily secondary to an active infectious process. Finally, in patients to whom "immunotherapy" is given after cessation of chemotherapy, appropriate control studies are needed before one can attribute enhancement of immune response to the "immunotherapy"; the enhancement might simply be the result of immunological rebound.

References

1. Simone, J., Aur, R. J. A., Hustu, H. O., Pinkel, D.: " Total Therapy" studies of acute lymphocytic leukemia in children. Current results and prospects for cure. Cancer (Philad.) (in press).
2. Pinkel, D., Hernandez, K., Borella, L., Holton, C., Aur, R. J. A., Samoy, G., Pratt, C.: Drug dosage and remission duration in childhood lymphocytic leukemia. Cancer (Philad.) 27, 247—256 (1971).

3. GEORGE, P., HERNANDEZ, K., HUSTU, O., BORELLA, L., HOLTON, C., PINKEL, D.: A study of "total therapy" of acute lymphocytic leukemia in children. J. Pediat. **72**, 399—408 (1968).
4. AUR, R. J. A., SIMONE, J. V., HUSTU, H. O., WALTERS, T., BORELLA, L., PRATT, C., PINKEL, D.: Central nervous system therapy and combination chemotherapy of childhood lymphocytic leukemia. Blood **37**, 272—281 (1971).
5. AUR, R. J. A., SIMONE, J. V., HUSTU, H. O., VERZOSA M. S.: A comparative study of central nervous system irradiation and intensive chemotherapy early in remission of childhood acute lymphocytic leukemia. Cancer (Philad.) **29**, 381—391 (1972).
6. AUR, R. J. A., HUSTU, H. O., VERZOSA, M. S., WOOD, A., SIMONE, J. V.: Two forms of "prophylactic" central nervous system (CNS) therapy in childhood acute lymphocytic leukemia. Proc. Amer. Ass. Cancer Res. **13**, 54 (1972).
7. BORELLA, L., WEBSTER, R. G.: The immunosuppressive effects of long-term combination chemotheraphy in children with acute leukemia in remission. Cancer Res. **31**, 420—426 (1971).
8. BORELLA, L., GREEN, A., WEBSTER, R. G.: Immunological rebound after cessation of long-term chemotherapy in acute leukemia. Blood **40**, 42—51 (1972).
9. BORELLA, L., GREEN, A. A.: Sequestration of PHA-responsive cells (T-lymphocytes) in the bone marrow of leukemic children undergoing immunosuppressive therapy. J. Immunol. **109**, 927—932 (1972).
10. GREEN, A. A., BORELLA, L.: Immunologic rebound after cessation of long-term chemotherapy in acute leukemia. II. *In vitro* responses to phytohemagglutinin and antigens by peripheral blood and bone marrow lymphocytes. Blood (in press).

Recent Results in Acute Leukemias at the Hospital Saint-Louis

J. Bernard, M. Boiron, Cl. Jacquillat, and M. Weil

Hôpital Saint-Louis, Paris/France

In this presentation, we shall briefly comment on some illustrations of our recent results in acute leukemias.

A. Results in ALL in Children

Table 1 summarizes the results of induction treatment in 367 children with ALL who were treated from 1964 to 1968 at the Hospital St. Louis: 205 children were treated with the combination of prednisone and vincristine, and 162 with the combination of prednisone and weekly doses of vincristine and daunorubicin. The rate of CR is better with prednisone, vincristine and daunorubicin than with prednisone and vincristine, while the number of deaths in induction is similar for both types of treatment; however, there was no randomization and no conclusion can be readed.

Table 2 shows the causes of death in induction. With better precautions concerning adjustment of doses in tumoral forms with hyperleukocytosis, and with the help of allopurinol, uratic nephropathy should be now avoided.

Of more concern, perhaps, are deaths in hematological complete remission, as shown in Table 3. With each protocol that we used, in spite of differences in maintenance and in the reinduction regimen, the death rate in remission is nearly 10%. Pneumopathy is obviously the most frequent cause of death here.

Table 1. Results of induction. St. Louis Paris 1964—1968

Induct. regimen	Pred + Vin 02-04 La Paris A.L.G.B. 6601 6801 A.	Pred + Vin + Daun 6606 A.L.G.B. 6801 B.	Total
No. patients	205	162	367
Deaths in induction	6 (3%)	7 (4%)	13
Failures	20 (10,5%)	2 (3,1%)	22
CR	179	150	329
Rate of CR	87,3% ± 4,6%	92,6% ± 4,3%	89,6%
	$p < 004$		

Table 2. Causes of death in induction

	Pred + Vin	Pred + Vin + Daun
Sepsis	3	3
Meningeal bleeding	1	3
Uratic nephropathy	2	1
Total	6/205	7/162

Table 3. Causes of death in hematol. CR (< 20 years)

	02-04	6606	A.L.G.B. 6601	A.L.G.B. 6801	Total
Pneumopathy	4	4	2	5	15
Sepsis			1		1
Varicella	1	2		2	5
Hepatitis		2			2
Lumbar punct. acc.	2				2
Cardiac toxicity				1	1
Car accident		1			1
Unknown			2	8	2
Total	7	9	5	113	29
No. initial CR	76 9%	90 10%	50 10%	7%	329 8,8%

Table 4. Chronology of fatal complications in complete remission

Months	Pneumopathy	Sepsis	Varicella	Hepatitis	Lumbar punct. acc.	Cardiac toxicity	Car accident	Unknown	Total
0—3	7	1	3						11
3—6	3			1				2	6
6—9	3			1					4
9—12			1						1
12—18	1								1
18—24			1						1
24—36						2	1		3
36—48									
48	1						1		2
Total	15	1	5	2	2	2	2	2	29/329

Table 4 shows the chronology of fatal complications in remission. They occur mainly during the first year when drug administration is heaviest. Lumbar puncture accidents are exceptional and always occur in children who have had many previous intrathecal methotrexate doses: although the mechanism of neurotoxicity is still unknown, the role of the chemical substance which acts as preservative for methotrexate cannot be ruled out. Cardiac death was observed in a girl who received 34 mg/kg of daunorubicin over 32 months. Let us recall that in protocol 06 LA 66, where large doses were given over a long period of time, no accident was observed. Duration of treatment as well as total amount of drug is an important factor in the cardiac toxicity of daunorubicin.

Fig. 1 compares the duration of complete hematological remissions and of complete remissions, including meningeal ones, for the protocols 02 LA 64, 04 LA 65, 06 LA 66.

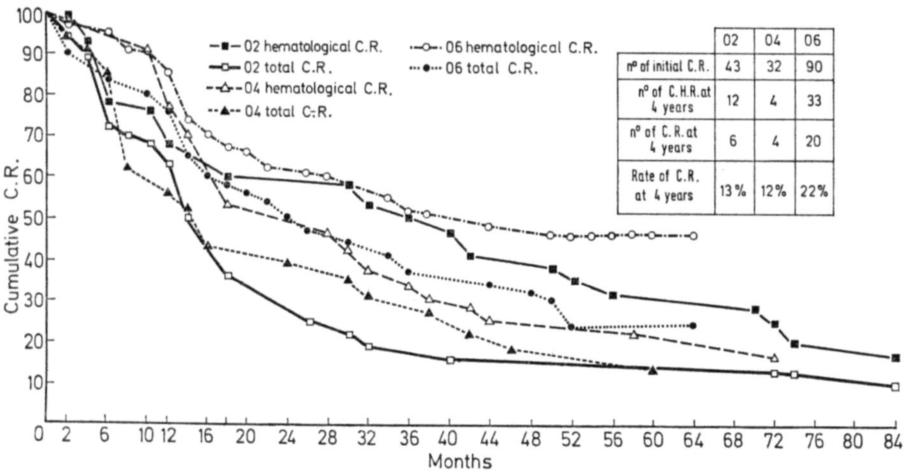

Fig. 1

In protocol 02 LA 64 where meningeal prophylaxis was belated and minimal, there is a big difference between the two categories of remissions; in protocol 04 LA 65, this difference is slight; in protocol 06 LA 66, in spite of early and frequent intrathecal methotrexate doses, there is still a significant difference between hematological complete remission and complete remission; this difference emphasizes by contrast the advantage of Pinkel's approach of skull irradiation. However, in our experience, a small group of patients who had early meningeal relapses have not developed hematological relapse after 4 to 6 years; therefore, one cannot always predict that a hematological relapse will follow a meningeal one.

It should be noted that 06 LA 66 results are better than those of the previous protocols. The cumulative rate of *complete hematological remission* at 4 years is 50%.

The cumulative rate of *complete remission* at 4 years is 22%, while it is 12% and 13% for protocols 02 and 04.

B. Long-Term Survivals

These advances, however, would be meaningless were they not associated with the hope of long-term survival. We have recently studied 214 patients whose survival exceeds 4 years (Table 5). Fig. 2 shows that cures may be hoped for only in patients who had no hematological nor meningeal relapse during the first four years.

Table 5. Survival for 4 or more years

	Children	Adults	Total
ALL	181	13	194
AML	8	14	22
Total	187	27	216

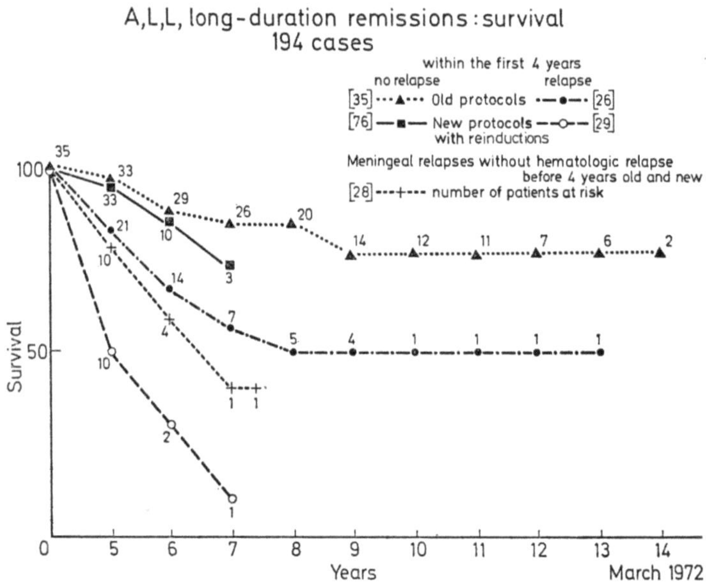

Fig. 2

C. Results in Acute Granulocytic Leukemias

In AML, daunorubicin, or combinations including it, achieves nearly 50% complete remissions; the median duration of these remissions is still poor (8 months) although some patients have long-term survival.

By contrast the relatively long duration of complete remission in acute promyelocytic leukemia (median 27 months) where the rate of complete remissions is 50% may be stressed. It illustrates the relationship between sensitivity to a given drug and the specific properties of a given cytological variety of leukemias. The unusual number of long-term survivals in a form of acute leukemia, the fulminant course of which was the main characteristic a few years ago, gives us reason to hope.

A New Agent Active in the Treatment of Acute Myeloblastic Leukemia 22 050 RP

CL. JACQUILLAT, M. WEIL, M-F. GEMON, V. IZRAEL, M. BOIRON, and J. BERNARD

Hôpital Saint-Louis, Paris/France

This report concerns our preliminary clinical experience in 44 cases of acute myeloblastic leukemia with 22 050 RP (Fig. 1), the benzoyl-hydrazone chlorhydrate of daunorubicin (DNR). Among the semi-synthetic derivatives of DNR, 22 050 RP in L 1210 leukemia has a better therapeutic index than DNR (10 to 15 for 22 050 RP, 5 to 10 for DNR). Moreover, it is 50% less toxic than DNR and 75% less toxic than adriamycin [3].

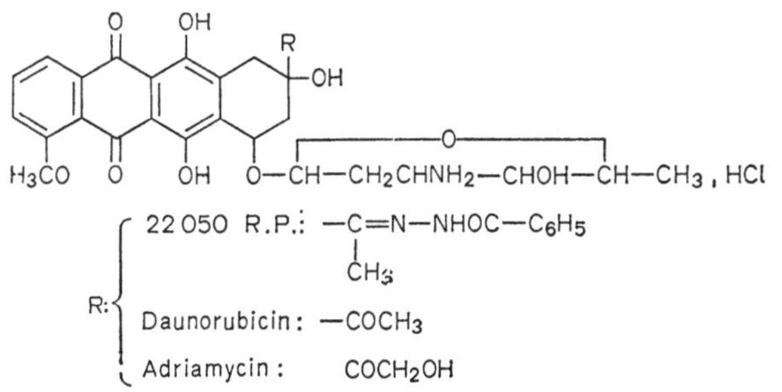

Fig. 1. Structures of 22 050 RP, daunorubicin, and adriamycin

Patients and Methods

In these 44 patients, the diagnosis of AML was ascertained by the usual panoptic stain, by the cytochemistry (PAS-negative, peroxydase positive): in 3 cases however both reactions were negative. The distribution of the cases is showed in Table 1 and Fig. 2.

Twenty patients in the first evolutive period had received no prior treatment. Four patients in the first evolutive period and all patients in relapse had received previously DNR alone (2 cases) or in combination with cytoxan, ara-c and L-asparaginase (protocole 09-71) (21 cases). The four patients in first evolutive period previously treated were resistant to these drugs.

Table 1. Distribution of cases of AML treated by 22 050 RP

	First attack		1st relapse	2nd relapse	Total
	No prior treatment	Prior treatment			
Children	5	2	6	2	15
Adults	15	3	10	1	29
Total	20	5	16	3	44

The daily dose of drug (3 to 5 mg/kg) was dissolved in 10 ml of saline and injected into the tubing of 200 ml of saline. Daily doses were repeated for 4 to 7 days in order to attain the total dose of 20 mg/kg. Blood counts were done daily. Bone marrow tests were performed on the days 5, 10, 15, 20 and 25. Bone marrow aplasia is generally noted from the day 10. If at this time blastic cells persist in the bone marrow, although white cells may be low (WBC 1000/mm^3), 1, 2 or 3 additional doses of 22 050 RP (3 mg/kg) are given according to the rate of persistent blastic cells (1 dose if blastic cells are between 10 an 20%; 2 doses for 20 and 50% blastic cells, and 3 doses for more than 50% blastic cells).

During the aplasic phase, antibiotic treatment was essential in all our patients. Platelet transfusions were given to all patients; white blood cell transfusions from CML donors were given to 17 patients.

Results

Overall Results

Our criteria of response are those of acute leukemia group B [2]. Complete remission implies ratings M1 — H1 —P1 — S1.

However, in some cases the score was M1 — H2 — P1 — S1 at the end of the induction phase because of belated complete recovery of hemopoiesis. Some days later, on maintenance phase, disease status A was attained. Results are summarized in Table 2.

Table 2. Results obtained with 22 050 RP in induction treatment for AML + one case eliminated (the treatment was stopped on day 2)

	1st attack No treatment		Prior treatment		1st relapse		2nd relapse		Total
	children	adults	children	adults	children	adults	children	adults	
Complete remission	3	9	1	—	2	5	—	—	20
Partial remission	1	1	—	—	—	—	—	—	2
Failure	—	3	1	2	4	4	2	—	16
Death in induction	1	2	—	1	—	1	—	1	6
Total	5	15	2	3	6	10	2	1	44+(45,4%)

The overall rate of complete remission was 45% (20 out of 44 patients).

In the 20 patients in first attack without prior treatment 12 complete remissions were achieved (60% complete remission).

In the 16 patients treated for the first relapse, 7 complete remissions were achieved and there were 8 failures. The 3 patients in other relapses were in the terminal phase of their disease and their condition was poor: two were resistant to 22 050 RP, one died in aplasia. The results, according to age and sex, are shown in Fig. 2.

There are no differences between children (under 20 years) and adults. Two complete remissions were achieved in patients more than 60 years old.

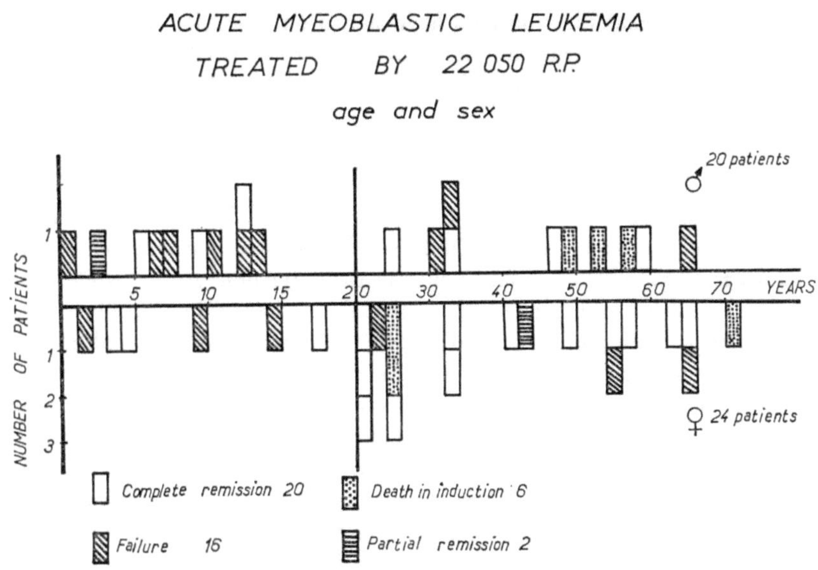

Fig. 2

Analytical Results

a) Complete remission (CR): the median dose necessary to achieve complete remission was 23 mg/kg; in 5 patients 15 mg/kg was sufficient whereas in 1 patient more than 30 mg/kg was necessary. These doses were delivered within a period of time extending from 10 to 30 days showing that belated doses of 22 050 RP are still active.

The median day when the complete disappearance of blastic cells and the return of normal hemopoietic cells were noted, was day 25. However, in most cases, bone marrow remained still hypoplastic and the return of platelets to normal counts was delayed so that the criteria for complete remission were fulfilled between day 30 and day 40.

b) Failure and death in induction. Deaths in induction were noted during the bone marrow aplasia induced by the first course of drug. Among failures, resistance was complete in one case—no decrease of bone marrow leukemic infiltration—. In other cases resistance consisted in blastic regeneration after a more or less marked aplasia induced by one course of 22 050 RP (8 cases) or by more than one course (8 cases).

Duration of CR

After completion of CR, patients receive a maintenance treatment of 6-mercaptopurine (90 mg/m²/d/p.o.), methyl-GAG (350 mg/m²/W/I.M.) and reinduction of ara-C (40 mg/m²/d/5d./s.c./every month). It is too early yet to have an idea of the duration of CR, which at present exceeds 4 months in 4 patients.

Toxicity

The drug was well tolerated: rashes (3 patients), nausea or vomiting (3 patients) and diarrhea (6 patients) were however noted; alopecia was constant. Hitherto routine hepatic and renal function tests have shown no alteration ascribable to the treatment. In one patient with a history of myocardial trouble, 22 050 RP was stopped after two doses for a sinusal tachycardy (160) without any other ECG changes.

Discussion

22 050 RP is an active drug in AML since it induced CR in 20/44 patients. Its chemical structure is close to that of DNR which suggested a comparison between these two drugs (Fig. 3). They differ mainly in their dynamic aspect: while daunorubicin was stricking in its drastic action, so that the necessary dose has given within the shortest possible period of time [3, 6], 22 050 RP may be administered in a more fractionated way over a longer period of time, allowing the dose to be adjusted to each patient. It is to be noted that regeneration is also progressive with some maturation disorders (however, it is M 1 according to international criteria) during two weeks or more and with a prolonged and moderated cytopenia. It has been proved that resistance occurs early with DNR [4] mainly if the treatment is intermittent. This resistance seems delayed with 22 050 RP, although this point has not yet been investigated by biochemical studies. Few patients died during the aplasic phase; this may be explained by progress in supportive therapy and by the better availability of white blood cell transfusions but also by the fact that 22 050 RP is easier to handle than DNR. Being active in AML as well as in ALL, where we obtained 55% complete remissions in relapses, 22 050 RP, having less marked toxicity than DNR, appears to be as a promising drug. However, more time is needed before its superiority over DNR can be regarded as proved.

Comparison between 22050 R.P. and D.N.R.

	22 050 R.P.	D.N.R.
Type of action	Progressive	Drastic
Median dose to ind. C.R.	25 mg/kg 750 mg/m²	10 mg/kg 300 mg/m²
Median day of C.R.	30	30
Main cause of FAILURE	RESISTANCE	APLASIA

Fig. 3. Comparison between 22 050 RP and D.N.R.

References

1. Bonadonna, G., Monfardini, S., de Lena, M., Fossati-Bellani, F.: Clinical evaluation of Adriamycin, a new antitumor antibiotic. Brit. med. J. **3**, 5669, 503—506 (1969).
2. Ellison, R. R., Holland, J. F., Weil, M., Jacquillat, Cl., Boiron, M., Bernard, J., Sawitsky, A., Rosner, F., Gussoff, B., Silver, R. T., Karanas, A., Cuttner, J., Spurr, C. L., Hayes, D. M., Blom, J. L., Leone, L. A., Haurani, F., Kyle, R., Hutchison, J. L., Forcier, L. J., Moon, J. H.: Arabinosyl Cytosine: A useful agent in the treatment of acute leukemia in adults. Blood **4**, 507—523 (1968).
3. Maral, R., Julou, L., Ganter, P., Populaire, P., Pasquet, J., Pascal, S., Detaille, J. Y., Delsques, M., Myon, J., Mondot, S.: Laboratoire de Recherches de la Société des Usines Chimiques Rhône Poulenc Vitry-sur-Seine (94). Etude de l'activité antitumorale et de la toxicité du 22 050 RP (Communication personnelle).
4. Skeel, R. T., Bertino, J. R., Creasey, W. A.: Clinical and pharmacologic studies with Daunorubicin in acute leukemia (Abstract). Clin. Res. **18**, 2476 (1970).
5. Weil, M., Glidewell, O., Jacquillat, Cl., Boiron, M., Bernard, J., Holland, J. F.: Studies of various doses and schedules of administration of Daunorubicin in acute granulocytic leukemia (analysis of A.L.G.B. protocols 6706 and 6706 A.) (in press).

Comparative Results Obtained in the Treatment of Acute Lymphoid Leukemia, Acute Myeloid Leukemia, and Acute Monocytoid Leukemia

L. Schwarzenberg [1], G. Mathé [1], P. Pouillart [1], R. Weiner [2], M. Hayat [1], J. L. Amiel [1], C. Jasmin [1], C. Rosenfeld [1], F. De Vassal [1], M. Schneider [3], and A. Cattan [4]

Acute lymphoid leukemia (ALL) and acute myeloid leukemia (AML) patients have been treated in our Institute according to different therapeutic principles (Fig. 1). *In ALL* we have tried to *induce remission with chemotherapy*, then applied *complementary cell-reducing systemic chemotherapy combined with CNS chemoradiotherapy* in order to reduce by three or four orders of magnitude the number of leukemic cells left by induction chemotherapy; finally we have submitted the patients to *active immunotherapy*, which is a combination of the injection of allogeneic leukemic cells and the administration of systemic adjuvants of immunity such as BCG [1, 2].

In AML, we have tried to induce remission and, when it is obtained, give *maintenance chemotherapy* until relapse.

In ALL, the incidence of so-called first "complete" remission (Table 1) is high if prednisone (PDN) and vincristine (VCR) are combined (93%). The triple combination of PDN, VCR and daunorubicin (DRB) that we gave in one trial (with 100% remission in children) was abandoned because of the high toxicity of DRB. At present

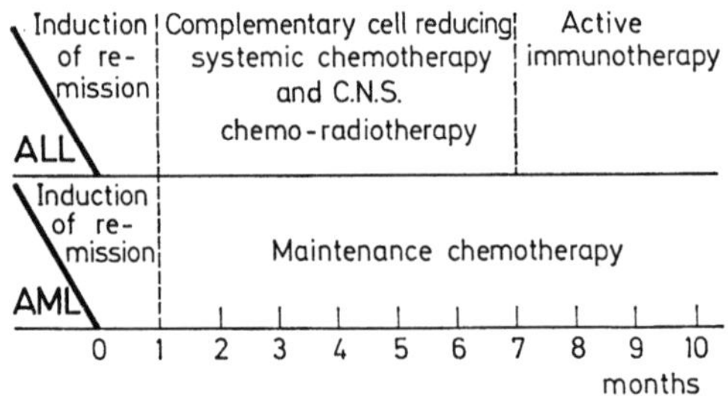

Fig. 1. Principles of our treatment protocols in acute lymphoid leukemia and in acute myeloid leukemia

[1] Institut de Cancérologie et d'Immunogénétique, Hôpital Paul-Brousse, Villejuif/France.
[2] Division of Medical Oncology, Harvard University, Medical School, Boston, MA/USA.
[3] C.A.C., Nice/France and
[4] C.R.L.C., Reims/France.

Table 1. Acute lymphoid leukemia. Incidences of first "complete" remission. (Experience of our services)

	ALL	AML	AMoL
PDN	58%		
DRB	25%	18%	
ADM	36%	33%	1/3
ASP	43%	20%	
CAR	25%	18%	1/2
MGGH		33%	
9ME		20%	
EPE			2/4
(VP 16)		25%	1/2
PDN+VCR+DRB	Children: 100% All ages: 85%		
PDN+VCR	All ages: 93%		
id. followed by ADM if failure	All ages: 98%		
CAR+THG		15%	
CAR+DRB		20,5%	

we use PDN and VCR and give adriamycine (ADM) only when PDN+VCR fails to induce remission. This reduces the use of a highly aplastic drug to a few patients who can be kept in our isolation unit [3, 4]. Therefore, there have been no deaths with the induction protocol.

Our results with AML have been much less encouraging. We find no difference in the incidence of "complete" remission induced by cytosine arabinoside (CAR), DRB, L-asparaginase (ASP), 9-methoxyellipticine (9-ME): about 20% for these four drugs; or by ADM, methyl-glyoxal(bis)-guanyl-hydrazone (MGGH) (33%); or by combinations DRB+VCR+PDN (25%); of CAR+DRB (20.5%), of CAR+thioguanine (THG) (15%).

In acute monocytoid leukemia (AMoL) the incidence of "complete" remission is as follows: 1 out of 3 with ADM; 1 out of 2 with CAR; 2 out of 4 with 4′-demethyl-epipodophyllotoxine -β-D-ethylidene-glucoside (VP-16-213) (EPE) [5] (Fig. 2); 1 out of 2 with the triple combination PDN+VCR+DRB.

Considering the actuarial curves for the duration of the first "complete" remission (Fig. 3), we have confirmation of the poor results obtained in AML: not only are the complete remissions notably few in number but they are short in duration, the median duration being 1.5 months and the longest 16 months. There is no difference according to age. On the contrary, even with a *geometrical representation of the time scale*, the Fig. 3 shows the very exciting overall results obtained in ALL: the median duration of the first "complete" remission is about 16 months and the curve is broken to form a plateau with no relapse between 32 months and about 5 years. We think it is not unreasonable to consider this plateau as the *statistical expression of "cure expectancy":* as can be seen on this figure, there is no great difference according to age and this cure expectancy group comprises about 33% of the patients.

As far as the toxic cost of our treatment schedule is concerned (Table 2), it is noticeably high (more than 18%) for a poor therapeutic result in AML; it is nil in

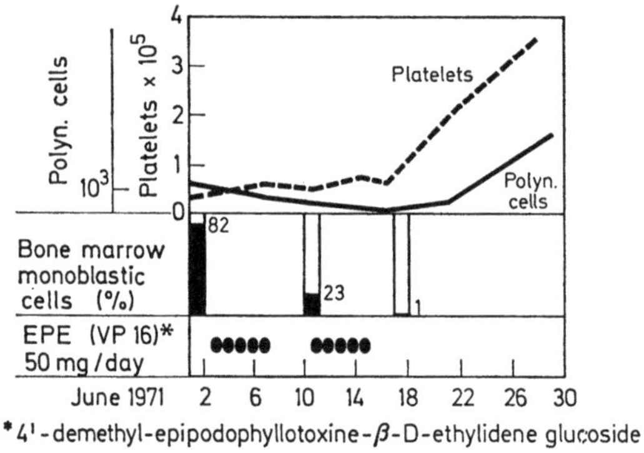

Fig. 2. Acute myelomonocytoid leukemia: the myeloblasts were much reduced after a CAR course, while the monoblasts increased. The latter disappeared after a VP 16213 course

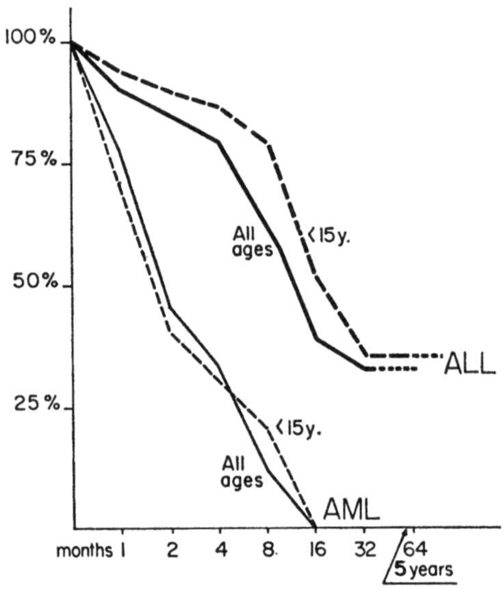

Fig. 3. Actuarial curves of the duration of first remission

Table 2. Toxic cost during "induction" and first remission

	Remission induction chemotherapy		Complementary cell reducing chemotherapy		Active immunotherapy	
ALL	Lethal	Non lethal toxicity	Lethal	Non lethal toxicity	Lethal	Non lethal toxicity
	0	0	0	4 paraplegias	0	0
AML	13%		5%			

ALL where we have experienced no mortality. Our lack of toxicity in ALL must be emphasized in the light of the 16% incidence of therapeutic deaths reported by some groups [6] and the higher figure mentioned orally by others (GLIDEWELL, MIESCHER). We take this to be an argument in favor of immunotherapy.

We regret the occurrence of paraplegia in 4 patients during their intrathecal chemotherapy; we suspect this is due to additives in methotrexate and cytosine arabinoside or their diluents. With the elimination of the additives we expect this complication to disappear [7].

In Table 3 we see the incidence of subsequent remissions obtained after patients have relapsed: the more relapses, the poorer the prognosis. This indicates that ALL represents a medical emergency that must be treated as early as possible by specialized centers equipped to give the most effective therapy and the most up-to-date supportive care.

The results of our trials can be illustrated by the actuarial curve of the cumulative duration of survival (Fig. 4): our survival data are poor for AML and are independent of age. They are remarkable for ALL. We recall that MATHÉ *et al.* [8] have shown the correlation of prognosis with the cytological variety of the disease, and that more

Table 3. Other remissions

	ALL	AML
2nd perceptible phase (PP)	87,5%	23%
3rd PP	58%	2/6
4th PP	34%	

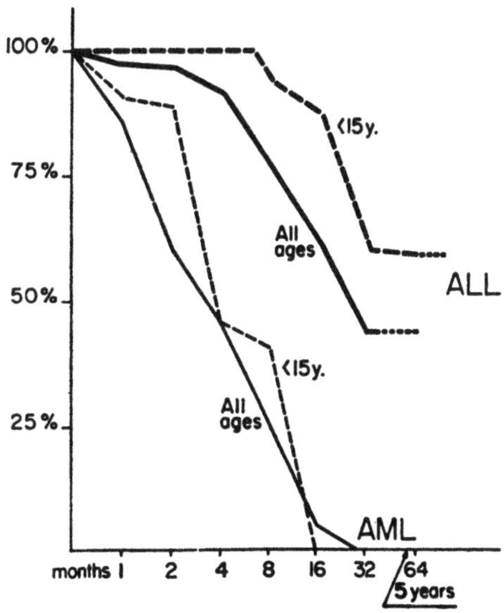

Fig. 4. Actuarial curves of the duration of cumulative survival

than 90% of the patients with the microlymphoblastic type are alive after 5 years. Considering the overall results in ALL, we see that the median of survival is 32 months for all ages, with a plateau for more than 40% of the patients. Here there is a difference according to age: for patients younger than 15, the actuarial curve of cumulative survival has not yet fallen to 50% and we do not know the median. We hope that the median will remain incalculable and the plateau will remain at 60%.

These are our actuarial results. They can be improved without any scientific progress, but with logistic progress. We must receive the patient at the very beginning of his disease.

References

1. MATHÉ, G.: Immunothérapie active de la leucémie L 1210 appliquée après la greffe tumorale. Rev. franç. Étud. clin. biol. **13**, 881—883 (1968).
2. MATHÉ, G.. POUILLART, P., LAPEYRAQUE, F.: Active immunotherapy of L 1210 leukemia applied after the graft of tumor cells. Brit. J. Cancer **23**, 814—824 (1969).
3. MATHÉ, G., FORESTIER, P.: Un outil moderne de la recherche médicale française; l'Institut de Cancérologie et d'Immunogénétique. Intrications de la recherche expérimentale et clinique. Conditionnement hyposeptique des animaux et malades. Techn. hosp. **20**, 47 (1965).
4. SCHNEIDER, M., SCHWARZENBERG, L., AMIEL, J. L., CATTAN, A., SCHLUMBERGER, J. R., HAYAT, M., DE VASSAL, F., JASMIN, C., ROSENFELD, C., MATHÉ, G.: Three year experience of the clinical use of a pathogen-free isolation unit. Brit. Med. J. **1**, 836 (1969).
5. MATHÉ, G., AMIEL, J. L., SCHWARZENBERG, L., SCHNEIDER, M., WEINER, R., POUILLART, P., HAYAT, M., DE VASSAL, F., JASMIN, C., ROSENFELD, C.: Clinical screening of VM26 and VP16213 in leukemias, hematosarcomas and solid tumors. Cancer, 1973, in press.
6. SIMONE, J. V., HOLLAND, E., JOHNSON, W.: Fatalities during remissions of childhood leukemia. Blood **39**, 759—770 (1972).
7. POUILLART, P., SCHWARZENBERG, L., SCHNEIDER, M., AMIEL, J. L., MATHÉ, G.: Les méningites lymphoblastiques: Incidence, prévention et traitement. Nouv. Presse Méd. **1**, 387—390 (1972).
8. MATHÉ, G., POUILLART, P., STERESCU, M., AMIEL, J. L., SCHWARZENBERG, L., SCHNEIDER, M., HAYAT, M., DE VASSAL, F., JASMIN, C., LAFLEUR, M.: Subdivision of classical varieties of acute leukemia. Correlation with prognosis and cure expectancy. Europ. J. clin. biol. Res. **16**, 554—560 (1971).

Preliminary Results of a Trial on Acute Myeloid Leukemia Comparing the Effect of Cytosine Arabinoside, the Combination of Cytosine Arabinoside and Thioguanine and the Combination of Cytosine Arabinoside and Daunorubicine

"Leukemia and Hematosarcoma" Cooperative Group *
of the European Organisation for Research on the Treatment of Cancer
(E.O.R.T.C.)

This paper records the preliminary results of a cooperative trial at a number of European centers in the treatment of acute myeloid leukemia (AML). It was carried out under the auspices of the Leukemia and Hematosarcoma Group of the European Organization for Research on Treatment of Cancer (E.O.R.T.C.).

Patients of all ages whose clinical state, peripheral blood and bone marrow findings were those of AML were admitted to the trial. Admission was confined to those who had had no previous treatment and whose bone marrow test at a single reference center, in this case Professor MATHÉ's laboratory, confirmed the diagnosis of AML or acute myelomonocytoid leukemia. On admission to the center and as soon as the diagnosis was made, the patient was randomized following instructions from the central organization. Slides were then dispatched and if the diagnosis was confirmed, the patient remained in the trial. In this way there was no delay in treatment. The patients were randomized into three groups for treatment, and randomization took into account age, percentage of typically granulocytic blasts and of blast presenting a "lymphoblast-like" aspect. The three treatment groups are shown in Table 1.

---

* Chairman: J. S. MALPAS (London). Secretary: M. HAYAT (Villejuif). Councillor: G. MATHÉ (Villejuif). Members: *Allemagne:* R. GROSS (Köln-Lindenthal), H. HEIMPEL, M. DIETRICH (Ulm), H. LÖFFLER (Gießen), P. OBRECHT (Freiburg im Breisgau); *Belgique:* C. CAUCHIE, Y. KENIS, R. MAURUS, J. P. NAETS, P. STRYCKMANS, H. TAGNON (Bruxelles), J. M. ANDRIEN, P. CONINX, J. HUGUES (Liège), P. PEETERMANS (Antwerpen); *Espagne:* M. RIBAS-MUNDO, C. FERRAN, J. ESTAPÉ (Barcelone); *France:* A. BERNADOU, G. BILSKI-PASQUIER, C. M. BLANC, J. BOUSSER, J. DEBRAY, M. KRÜLIK, R. ZITTOUN (Paris), A. CATTAN (Reims), J. CHAUVERGNE, B. HOERNI, G. SIMON (Bordeaux), D. FIERE, L. REVOL, J. J. VIALA (Lyon), PH. FRANÇOIS (Clermont-Ferrand), M. HAYAT, G. MATHÉ, L. SCHWARZENBERG (Villejuif), G. MAYER, S. MAYER, R. WAITZ (Strasbourg). H. PIGUET (Rouen); *Grande Bretagne:* T. J. MCELWAIN (Sutton), M. T. SHAW, J. S. MALPAS (London); *Hollande:* J. F. CLETON (Amsterdam), F. ELKERBOUT, B. SPECK (Leiden), C. HAANEN (Nijmwegen), H. KERKHOFS, C. H. W. LEEKSMA (La Haye), W. F. STENFERT-KROESE (Rotterdam); *Irlande:* J. B. HEALY (Dublin); *Italie:* L. BUSSI, D. CIPRIANI, A. PENSABENE (Milano), M. BACCARANI, S. TURA (Bologna), N. NIGRO, E. MADON, G. C. MUSSA (Torino).

Final results have been published in Biomedicine 18, 192 (1973).

Group 1 received cytosine arabinoside (CAR) alone for four days; group 2 received CAR and thioguanine (THG), the first drug being given for four days and the second for five days; group 3 received CAR for four days and was given daunorubicin (DRB) in addition on the first day. When the trial began, the recommended interval between courses was 10 days but shortly afterwards the time interval between courses was reduced and, hematological condition permitting, the interval was reduced to 5 or 6 days. The patients received at least three courses. A total of 194 patients were randomized and 167 of these were evaluated. It was important to see whether the three groups were comparable with regard to factors known to influence prognosis, such as age, sex, presence of bleeding manifestations, splenomegaly, thrombocytopenia and the peripheral blood count. There was no significant difference between the three groups, as shown in Table 2.

The groups were also comparable in the type of AML (Table 3).

When the patient finally achieved complete remission, as defined by return to a normal clinical state, normal peripheral blood film and a normal bone marrow, confirmed by the reference center, this was notified to the reference center. The analysis shows that there was no difference in remission rates between the three groups (Table 4). The rate of remission is rather low, at 18%, but other workers using exactly similar regimes have also experienced similarly low remission rates.

Table 1. E.O.R.T.C. trial in acute myeloid leukemia — May 1972. Treatment schedules

Induction	
Treatment 1	Cytosine arabinoside alone 75—100 mg/m² daily, days 1 to 4. i.v.
Treatment 2	Cytosine arabinoside 75—100 mg/m² daily, day 2 to day 5 i.v. Thioguanine 75—100 mg/m² daily, day 1 to day 5. orally
Treatment 3	Cytosine arabinoside 75—100 mg/m² daily, day 1 to day 4. i.v. Daunorubicin 60 mg/m² day 1 *only* i.v.

Table 2. E.O.R.T.C. trial in acute myeloid leukemia — May 1972. Comparison of groups: Clinical and hematological

Treatment	Number evaluated	Age	Sex M %	Sex F	Spleen+ %	Bleeding+ %	RBC $\times 10^5$	WBC $\times 10^2$	Pl $\times 10^3$	Bls $\times 10^2$
CAR alone	55	47.5	60	40	19	48	26.2	366	62	243
CAR+THG	53	47.4	53	47	15	47	30.4	270	62	127
CAR+DRB	55	51.5	53	47	21	45	27.0	274	77	157
		N. S.[a]	N. S.	N. S.	N. S.	N. S.	N. S.	N. S.	N. S.	N. S.

[a] N. S. = Not significant

Factors influencing remission have been examined in this series and have confirmed other studies in acute myeloid or myelomonocytoid leukemias. For example, older patients have done less well, and the rate of remission has been higher in those patients with classical myeloblastic leukemia and also the subgroup defined in our group as having had numbers of lymphoblast-like cells (see MATHÉ *et al.*). In this particular study we were unable to show any influence of the initial platelet count or blast cell count on the rate of induction of remission. There were some differences between the three groups in as far as only 2.7 courses of CAR + DRB were necessary to induce remission compared with three courses in the CAR + THG group, and 3.3 in the group treated with CAR alone. Survival of these patients was, of course, longer in those who achieved remission, but it was interesting that the group treated with CAR + DRB had a significantly better survival rate than the group treated with CAR + THG (Fig. 1) until the 18th month.

There was no major difference in toxic side effects as between the groups treated with CAR alone and CAR + DRB. In each group 13 patients succumbed, either from hemorrhage or infection during the course of treatment or in the 15 days following the course. Toxicity in the CAR + THG group was somewhat higher with 19 deaths.

The influence on survival of supportive therapy, such as facilities for platelet transfusions on demand, for isolation and white cell transfusion was investigated. It

Table 3. E.O.R.T.C. trial in acute myeloid leukemia — May 1972. Comparison of distribution of different cytological types

Bone marrow appearance	Treatment regime			
	CAR alone number %	CAR+THG	CAR+DRB	Total
Promyeloblastic	21—38%	18—35%	20—34%	59
Myeloblastic	14—26%	17—29%	14—26%	45
Promyelocytic	5— 8%	4— 8%	2— 3%	11
Myelomonocytoid	11—20%	8—16%	6—10%	25
All AML subvarieties with many lymphoblast-like cells	4— 8%	6—12%	13—25%	23

No significant difference between groups.

Table 4. E.O.R.T.C. trial in acute myeloid leukemia — May 1972. Remission rates in the three groups

	Number	C. R.	C. R. %
CAR alone	55	9	14.5 [a]
CAR+THG	53	8	15 [a]
CAR+DRB	55	12	21 [a]
Total	163	29	18

[a] No significant difference.

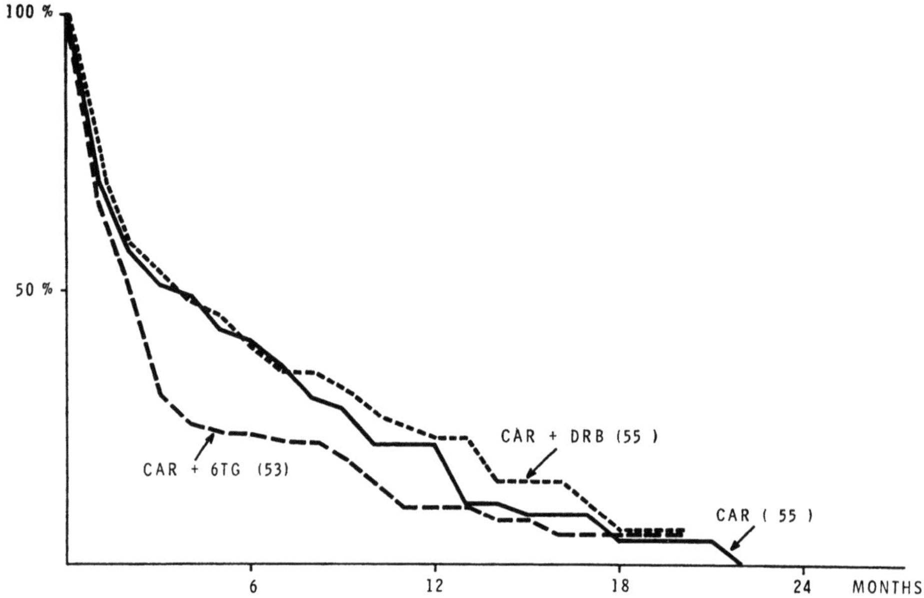

Fig. 1. Survival curves for different induction treatments

appeared that units able to produce this supportive therapy achieved 28% remission rates compared with 11.7% in other centers.

In conclusion, in this trial conducted in 27 different European centers, there was no difference in the frequency with which remission was obtained with the three treatment schedules employed. Age and cytological characteristics of the patients with AML have an important bearing on the frequency of remission, and patients going into remission survived longer.

References

Clarkson, B. D., Dowling, M. D., Gee, T. S., Burchenal, J. H.: Treatment of acute myeloblastic leukaemia. 1 vol., Bâle: Karger 1972.

Crowther, D., Bateman, C. J. T., Vartan, C. P., Whitehouse, J. M. A., Malpas, J. S., Hamilton-Fairley, G., Bodley Scott, R.: Combination chemotherapy using L-asparaginase in the treatment of acute myelogenous leukemia. Brit. med. J. 4, 513 (1970).

Henderson, E., Serpick, A., Leventhal, B., Henry, P.: Cytosine arabinoside infusions in adult and childhood acute myelocytic leukemia. Proc. Amer. Cancer Res. 9, 29 (1968).

Mathé, G., Pouillart, P., Hayat, M., Weiner, R., Steresco, M., Lafleur, M.: Classification and subclassification of acute leukemias correlated with clinical expression, therapeutic sensitivity and prognosis. In: Acute leukemias nomenclature, classification, clinical trials, methodology and actuarial results, vol. 1. Eds.: G. Mathé, P. Pouillart, L. Schwarzenberg. Berlin-Heidelberg-New York: Springer 1973.

Schwarzenberg, L., Mathé, G., Hayat, M., De Vassal, F., Amiel, J. L., Cattan, A., Schneider, M., Schlumberger, J. R., Rosenfeld C., Jasmin, C.: Essai de traitement des leucémies aiguës par la cytosine arabinoside selon la méthode de Skipper. Nouv. Rev. franç. Hémat. 9, 199 (1969).

*43 Nomenclature, Methodology and Results of Clinical Trials in Acute Leukemias (Symposium). Edited by G. MATHÉ, L. SCHWARZENBERG, P. POUILLART, Villejuif. Cloth DM 58,—; US $ 23.80

Special Supplement: Biology of Amphibian Tumors. Edited by M. MIZELL, New Orleans. Cloth DM 86,—; US $ 35.30

In Production

*44 GRUNDMANN, E., Münster: Special Topics in Carcinogenesis (Symposium)

45 KOLDOVSKY, P., Philadelphia: Carcinoembryonic Antigens

46 MATHÉ, G., WEINER, R., Villejuif: Investigation and Stimulation of Immunity in Cancer Patients (Symposium)

In Preparation

BOIRON, M.: The Viruses of the Leukemia-Sarcoma Complex

CAVALIERE, R., ROSSI-FANELLI, A., MONDOVI, B., and MORICCA, G.: Selective Heat Sensitivity of Cancer Cells

CONNORS, T. A., ROBERTS, J.: Platinum Coordination Complexes in Cancer Chemotherapy (Symposium)

GARATTINI, S., FRANCHI, G.: Chemotherapy of Cancer Dissemination: Methods and Results

GRUNDMANN, E.: Morphology and Cytochemistry of Carcinogenesis

KESSLER, I., AURELIAN, L.: Cancer of the Cervix: Problem, Progress, Prospects

LEVIN, A.: Human Tumour Immunology for Clinicians and Experimentalists

MATHÉ, G.: Immunotherapy of Cancer

MERKOW, L., SLIFKIN, M.: Oncogenic Simian Adenoviruses

OETTGEN, H. F.: Tumor Immunology

RICHTERS, A., SHERWIN, R.: Autochthonous Lymphocyte Interactions with Neoplastic and Non-neoplastic Human Cells

WEIL, R.: Biological and Structural Properties of Polyoma Virus and its DNA

MIX
Papier aus verantwortungsvollen Quellen
Paper from responsible sources
FSC® C105338

If you have any concerns about our products,
you can contact us on
ProductSafety@springernature.com

In case Publisher is established outside the EU,
the EU authorized representative is:
Springer Nature Customer Service Center GmbH
Europaplatz 3, 69115 Heidelberg, Germany

Printed by Libri Plureos GmbH
in Hamburg, Germany